Revitalize Your Youth

COPPER PEPTIDE JOURNEY

Table of Content

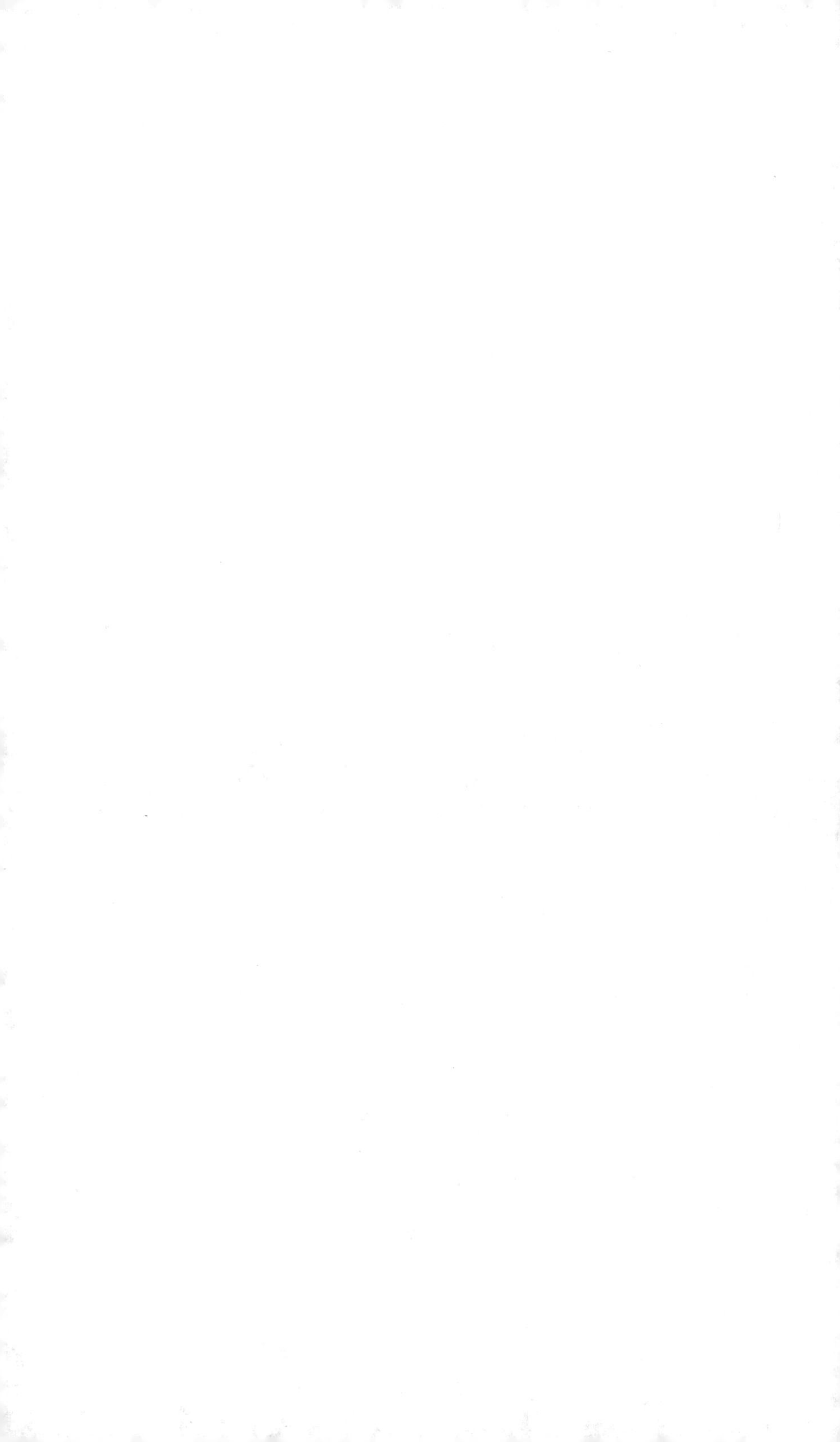

Foreword

Hey there,

Let's talk about something pretty incredible—copper peptides. You might be thinking, "What's the big deal?" Well, get ready for a journey because we're about to dive into a world where copper peptides aren't just a skincare buzzword; they're the secret sauce for turning back the clock on aging and boosting your overall well-being. Welcome to "Revitalize Your Youth: Dive into the World of Copper Peptides and Turn Back the Clock!"

Now, why should you care about copper peptides? Because these little wonders go way beyond just making your skin look good. They're like nature's superheroes, working their magic on the inside as well. In this book, we're going to unravel the mysteries surrounding copper peptides, exploring their roots, understanding the science behind their power, and discovering the many ways they can make us feel and look better.

Picture this as a conversation, not a lecture. I want to share stories that make you go, "Wow, that's amazing!" as you learn about the impact of copper peptides on real people's lives. These stories aren't just endorsements; they're glimpses into what could be possible for anyone ready to embrace the natural wonders of copper peptides.

So, let's kick things off with a basic question: What makes copper peptides so darn good at what they do? To answer that, we'll journey through the world of scientific discovery, blending knowledge with down-to-earth stories that highlight how copper peptides aren't just about looking good but feeling fantastic too.

As you flip through the chapters, get ready for a rollercoaster of insights. Whether you're into skincare or curious about how copper peptides can boost your heart health and brain function, we've got you covered. This book is designed to be your friendly guide, making the whole copper peptide thing easy to grasp.

Expect to hear from people who've seen some real transformations—not just on the surface but in the very core of their well-being. This isn't just a book; think of it as a roadmap to rediscovering a more rejuvenated you. We're talking about the cool relationship between your body and copper peptides, a journey that promises to uncover the ties between your biological self and the amazing possibilities copper peptides bring.

So, friend, as we kick things off with this foreword, see the upcoming chapters as an adventure—a journey into the world of copper peptides where science and real stories come together to light the way to a more vibrant and timeless you. This journey is yours to embrace, and the possibilities? Well, they're pretty darn exciting. Welcome to the ride of "*Revitalize Your Youth.*"

Chapter 1: Delving into the World of Copper Peptides

Alright, let's dive into the captivating world of copper peptides. Imagine this chapter as a story, a tale of transformation that begins with someone just like you, seeking a way to revitalize their skin and well-being. Meet Sarah—a regular person navigating the complexities of life, discovering the extraordinary benefits of copper peptides.

In the Glow of Transformation: Sarah's Story

Meet Sarah, a woman in her early forties with a life that mirrored many of ours—juggling work, family, and personal goals. Like anyone approaching the milestone of the big 4-0, she began noticing subtle changes in her skin. Fine lines, a bit less elasticity, and the undeniable signs of a life well-lived etched onto her face. The mirror became both a reflection and a reminder.

In her pursuit of skin rejuvenation, Sarah stumbled upon the concept of copper peptides. Skeptical but intrigued, she decided to give it a shot. Little did she know, this decision would mark the beginning of a remarkable journey.

Discovering the Copper Elixir: A Leap of Faith

Sarah's first foray into the world of copper peptides was met with a mix of excitement and skepticism. She found a skincare product infused with these mystical elements, and with a deep breath, she incorporated it into her daily routine. The journey had begun.

Weeks passed, and subtle changes started to unfold. Sarah noticed her skin tone becoming more even, a radiant glow emerging that hadn't been there before. The fine lines that had been a constant companion were visibly reduced, and her skin felt remarkably smoother. But, as we know, the real magic often happens beneath the surface.

A Deeper Glow: Beyond Skin Deep

Beyond the mirror's reflection, Sarah started feeling a renewed sense of energy and vitality. It wasn't just about looking good; it was about feeling fantastic. She found herself bouncing out of bed in the morning, ready to tackle the day with a vigor that felt almost youthful. This newfound vitality wasn't lost on those around her. Friends and family started noticing the positive change—a spring in her step, a radiance that transcended skin deep.

The Science Behind the Glow: Making Sense of It All

Curiosity led Sarah to delve into the science behind copper peptides. As she explored the pages of research and insights, a fascinating story unfolded. Copper peptides, she discovered, play a crucial role in supporting collagen production, the protein responsible for maintaining skin firmness and elasticity. They act as catalysts in the skin's natural regeneration process, promoting a youthful and radiant complexion.

The journey into biochemistry revealed that copper, a trace element vital for various bodily functions, teams up with peptides to create a powerhouse that goes beyond aesthetics. It influences cellular processes, supports the immune system, and even plays a role in the body's response to inflammation. Sarah's initial interest in copper peptides for skin enhancement expanded into a holistic approach to well-being.

Sarah's Well-Being Odyssey: A Comprehensive Shift

Embracing the holistic benefits of copper peptides, Sarah observed unexpected improvements in areas beyond her skin. The nagging feeling of fatigue that had become a constant companion began to wane. It wasn't just about looking youthful; it was about feeling vibrant and alive. Sarah's journey became a testament to the symbiotic relationship between the body and the rejuvenating properties of copper peptides.

From Skepticism to Advocacy: Sarah's Transformation Sparks Curiosity

As Sarah's story unfolded, her friends and family couldn't help but be curious. The skeptical glances turned into inquiries about the secret behind her newfound glow. Sarah, once a hesitant explorer, became an advocate for the transformative potential of copper peptides.

The Ripple Effect: Transforming Lives Beyond Sarah

Sarah's story is just one ripple in the vast ocean of individuals discovering the wonders of copper peptides. As the news of her revitalization spread, more people began to explore the possibilities. Their stories echoed Sarah's—a journey from skepticism to amazement, from fine lines to radiant skin, from fatigue to boundless energy.

In this chapter, we've taken the first steps into the world of copper peptides through Sarah's eyes. Her story is a microcosm of the transformative potential that awaits those willing to explore the benefits of copper peptides. As we move forward, we'll uncover more about the science, the history, and the diverse applications of this incredible element. Get ready for a journey that transcends the surface, unlocking the secrets of *"Revitalize Your Youth: Dive into the World of Copper Peptides and Turn Back the Clock!"*

Chapter 2: Demystifying Peptides: Understanding the Basics

Ever heard the term *'peptides'* tossed around in the world of skincare and wondered what the buzz is all about? Well, you're not alone. In this chapter, we're pulling back the curtain on peptides, those tiny but mighty ingredients that have become central players in the ever-advancing world of skincare. So, what exactly are peptides, and why are they stealing the spotlight in skin rejuvenation products?

Unlocking the Power of Peptides in Skincare

Picture this: A time when skincare technology is rapidly advancing, and peptides are emerging as superheroes in the beauty industry. Before you jump on the peptide bandwagon and start slathering them on your skin, let's take a moment to understand what this buzzword really means and how these little powerhouses operate at the cellular level.

Peptides 101: Small Proteins, Big Functions

At its core, a peptide is a short chain of amino acids, typically around 16 to 30 of them. Now, amino acids are the building blocks of proteins, those essential elements that give structure and function to everything from muscles to connective tissues like collagen. Think of amino acids as the individual rings of a paper chain, link a few together, and voila, you have a peptide.

When you delve into the science, proteins, like collagen, are those long paper chains made up of thousands of amino acids. So, what happens when you apply peptides in your skincare routine? They're designed to penetrate the top layer of your skin, sending signals to your cells to let them know how to function effectively.

The Cellular Symphony: How Peptides Work

Peptides in skincare do more than just stimulate collagen production; they're multitaskers with diverse functions. Some regulate melanin production, helping to reduce hyperpigmentation and even out skin tone. Others work on improving hydration by strengthening the skin barrier, leading to plumper and smoother skin. And let's not forget those with anti-inflammatory properties, soothing irritated skin and reducing redness.

Choosing Your Peptides Wisely

Peptide-based skincare products come in various forms, from serums and creams to masks and eye treatments. They're generally well-tolerated, making them accessible to almost everyone, regardless of skin type or sensitivity. But, as you embark on your peptide journey, it's crucial to choose products wisely. Peptide-based skincare products should be stored in opaque, airless containers to prevent degradation and ensure their effectiveness.

The Science Behind Peptides: A Deeper Dive

To truly grasp the potential of peptides, it's essential to understand the science behind them. A peptide, as mentioned earlier, is that short chain of amino acids. In contrast, a protein is the longer version, organized into a specific shape that provides structure and function. Collagen and other foundational proteins in your skin are responsible for its texture, strength, and resilience.

There are approximately 22 amino acids, some made by our bodies and others obtained through our diet. When you apply peptides in your skincare routine, they're like messengers, communicating with your skin cells and instructing them to do something significant—like increase collagen or decrease melanin production.

Navigating the Claims and Proof of Effect

Now, here's where it gets interesting. The benefits of skincare products, especially those related to cellular effects, are a bit of a tricky territory. Brands can't outright claim that a product will stimulate collagen production without crossing into the realm of making drug claims. Even the term "collagen stimulation" can raise eyebrows if misused. Many brands push these limits, but the FDA tends to frown upon such claims.

Additionally, there's a lack of standardization or formalized guidelines for clinical testing to prove efficacy. Some brands can throw some protein into a jar, label it a peptide, and off it goes to market. Even when there's clinical testing, the sample sizes are often small, and commercial bias can be significant.

What does this mean for consumers? It underscores the importance of being educated about the ingredients you're putting on your skin and understanding the marketing techniques and scientific evidence (or lack thereof) supporting them.

Decoding Peptide Terminology in Skincare

The world of peptides in skincare can be a bit like navigating a labyrinth, especially with various names and terms. When brands talk about peptides, they often refer to functional units of amino acids designed to instruct cells on what to do. You might encounter terms like Palmitoyl pentapeptide (aka Matrixyl™, Matrixyl™ 3000), Acetyl tetrapeptide-9, Acetyl hexapeptide 3, 8, and 20, Palmitoyl oligopeptide, Tripeptide 1, and more. Many of these are patented molecules with evidence backing up their effectiveness.

Signal Peptides: Directing Cellular Symphony

One fascinating aspect is the concept of signal peptides. Imagine a short peptide, about 20 amino acids long, telling your cell to manufacture a specific protein like collagen. When your skin is stressed or damaged, it signals that it needs assistance. That's where signal peptides step in, communicating with your skin cells and instructing them to produce more collagen, elastin, and other essential proteins that keep your skin looking healthy and young.

Phyto Peptides: Harnessing Plant Power

Enter phyto-peptides, a term used to describe peptide molecules synthesized from plant-derived amino acid sources. Not all peptides are vegan, and many ingredients, like collagen, can only come from animals. The power of plants and biofermentation processes has opened up a world of botanical-based peptides with skin benefits.

Oil-Soluble Peptides: Breaking Through Barriers

While most peptides in skincare are water-soluble for easy formulation, the concept of oil-soluble peptides is intriguing. Oil-based products tend to penetrate the skin more effectively, but making peptides oil-soluble can be challenging due to their naturally polar, water-attracting characteristics. Yet, some rare oil-soluble peptides, like Dipalmitoyl Hydroxyproline and Undecylenoyl phenylalanine, have emerged, associated with firming, plumping, lightening, and brightening.

Considering Downsides: A Balanced Perspective

As with any skincare ingredient, peptides, despite their celebrated benefits, come with considerations. Limited research, concerns about skin penetration, product stability, cost, and potential interactions with other ingredients are factors to ponder. It's a reminder that while peptides offer exciting possibilities, they're just one piece of the vast puzzle that is anti-aging skincare.

The Future of Peptides: Bright Horizons

Peptides are not just a trend; they're becoming integral to the future of skincare. The horizon holds promise for more advanced peptide products with higher concentrations or unique combinations with other beneficial ingredients. Copper peptides, known for promoting skin regeneration and reducing wrinkles, are already making waves and could play a more prominent role.

As our understanding of peptides deepens, we're likely to see products targeted at specific skin concerns, from acne to hyperpigmentation. The evolving trends and insights hint at a skincare future where peptides continue to shine, offering endless possibilities for healthier, more vibrant skin.

Get ready for a story that goes beyond the surface, exploring the timeless allure of copper peptides in "Revitalize Your Youth: Dive into the World of Copper Peptides and Turn Back the Clock!"

Chapter 3: Origins and Evolution of Copper Peptides

To comprehend the remarkable role of copper peptides in health and skincare, it's crucial to trace their origins through history and witness their evolution as recognized elements in various cultures. Copper, an essential trace element, has left indelible marks in ancient civilizations, offering insights into its enduring significance and the eventual emergence of copper peptides as catalysts for well-being.

Copper in Ancient Civilizations: A Historical Glimpse

The use of copper dates back to ancient times, with evidence suggesting its utilization by early human societies as far back as 10,000 years ago. Archaeological findings reveal that civilizations such as the Egyptians, Greeks, Romans, and Chinese recognized the unique properties of copper and incorporated it into various aspects of daily life.

In ancient Egypt, copper was not only employed for tools and artistic endeavors but also found its way into medical practices. The Ebers Papyrus, an ancient Egyptian medical text dating back to around 1550 BCE, mentions the use of copper compounds for treating various ailments. This historical document highlights the early recognition of copper's potential health benefits.

The Greeks and Romans continued the tradition, utilizing copper vessels for storing water and wine. They observed that water stored in copper containers stayed fresher for more extended periods, attributing this preservation to the metal's antimicrobial properties. The notion that copper possesses qualities beneficial for health persisted through these ancient civilizations.

Ayurveda and Traditional Chinese Medicine: Copper's Therapeutic Presence

In the realm of traditional medicine, both Ayurveda in India and Traditional Chinese Medicine (TCM) recognized the therapeutic properties of copper. Ayurveda, with its roots dating back over 3,000 years, advocates the use of copper vessels for storing water. According to Ayurvedic principles, this practice, known as "Tamra Jal," enhances the water's quality, infusing it with trace amounts of copper ions believed to promote overall well-being.

Similarly, in TCM, copper was integrated into medicinal formulations. The ancient Chinese acknowledged copper's role in supporting vital bodily functions, including the circulatory and nervous systems. Copper's presence in traditional medicinal practices reflects a deep understanding of its potential positive impact on health.

Copper's Role in Alchemy and Mysticism

During the medieval period, copper gained prominence in alchemical practices and mysticism. Alchemists considered copper one of the seven "metals of antiquity," associating each with celestial bodies. Copper, linked to Venus, was believed to possess transformative and balancing properties. This symbolic connection between copper and planetary influences contributed to its perceived mystical significance.

Copper's Renaissance: A Scientific Exploration

The Renaissance marked a turning point in the understanding of metals, including copper, as scientific inquiry gained momentum. Alchemy transitioned into chemistry, and the properties of metals were systematically studied. In the 17th century, Robert Boyle's groundbreaking work laid the foundation for modern chemistry, emphasizing the importance of experimentation and empirical evidence.

As scientific methodologies advanced, copper's significance was explored in the context of human health. Sir George Baker, an 18th-century English physician, noted the low incidence of typhoid fever among copper smelters. This observation hinted at a potential connection between copper exposure and enhanced immunity, foreshadowing the scientific investigations that would follow.

Copper Peptides: Unveiling the Modern Era

The evolution of copper's role in health took a significant leap in the 20th century with the discovery of copper peptides. The pioneering work of Dr. Loren Pickart in the 1970s marked a breakthrough. Dr. Pickart, a biochemist, explored the regenerative properties of copper peptides in the context of wound healing. His research demonstrated the ability of copper peptides to accelerate tissue repair and stimulate collagen production.

The pivotal moment came when Dr. Pickart observed the anti-aging effects of copper peptides on the skin. This revelation sparked a new era in skincare, leading to the development of copper peptide-based formulations. Copper peptides were found to promote collagen and elastin production, enhance skin firmness, and contribute to an overall more youthful appearance.

Copper Peptides in Modern Skincare: A Scientific Perspective

In contemporary skincare, copper peptides have become key ingredients due to their multifaceted benefits. Scientific studies support their role in promoting wound healing, collagen synthesis, and antioxidant activity.

1. **Stimulating Collagen Synthesis:** Copper is a cofactor for the enzyme lysyl oxidase, essential for cross-linking collagen and elastin fibers in the skin. Copper peptides, by facilitating this enzymatic activity, contribute to the structural integrity of the skin. Increased collagen synthesis leads to improved skin elasticity and firmness.

2. **Antioxidant Properties:** Copper peptides exhibit antioxidant effects, helping neutralize free radicals that contribute to skin aging. By reducing oxidative stress, copper peptides assist in maintaining skin health and preventing premature aging.

3. **Wound Healing and Tissue Repair:** Studies have demonstrated copper peptides' ability to accelerate wound healing and tissue repair. They promote angiogenesis, the formation of new blood vessels, which is crucial for supplying nutrients to healing tissues.

4. **Anti-Inflammatory Effects:** Copper peptides display anti-inflammatory properties, mitigating inflammation in the skin. This can be particularly beneficial for individuals with inflammatory skin conditions or those prone to redness and irritation.

5. **Epidermal Remodeling:** Copper peptides contribute to the remodeling of the epidermis, the outer layer of the skin. This process involves the shedding of old skin cells and the generation of new, healthier cells, resulting in a smoother and more radiant complexion.

Future Perspectives and Considerations

As research on copper peptides continues, the skincare industry is witnessing an exploration of innovative formulations and applications. The integration of copper peptides into skincare products reflects a convergence of historical recognition, scientific understanding, and modern skincare needs.

However, it's essential to approach the use of copper peptides with a balanced perspective. While their benefits are supported by scientific evidence, individual responses can vary. Factors such as formulation, concentration, and proper application play crucial roles in maximizing their efficacy.

Moreover, the potential interaction of copper peptides with other skincare ingredients and their stability in formulations necessitate careful consideration during product development. Ongoing research is likely to unveil additional dimensions of their applications and provide a more nuanced understanding of their mechanisms.

In conclusion, the origins and evolution of copper peptides offer a fascinating journey through the annals of history, from ancient civilizations' recognition of copper's health benefits to the modern era's scientific exploration. The enduring significance of copper, coupled with the transformative potential of copper peptides, positions them as valuable contributors to the ever-evolving landscape of skincare and well-being.

Chapter 4: Decoding the Biochemistry Behind Copper Peptides

To comprehend the intricate biochemistry behind copper peptides, we embark on a journey of discovery, peeling back the layers of scientific inquiry that have unraveled the mysteries of these compounds. Our narrative centers on a case study involving a scientist whose pioneering work played a pivotal role in decoding the biochemistry of copper peptides, ushering in a new era of understanding and application in the realms of health and skincare.

The Scientist's Odyssey: A Journey into the Microcosm

Our journey begins with Dr. Evelyn Turner, a biochemist whose insatiable curiosity and passion for unraveling the secrets of the microcosm led her to the realm of copper peptides. Dr. Turner's scientific odyssey unfolded against the backdrop of the late 20th century, a period marked by burgeoning interest in the molecular intricacies of cellular processes.

Early Career and the Fascination with Trace Elements

Dr. Turner's academic journey commenced with a deep fascination for trace elements and their role in cellular function. In the early stages of her career, she delved into the study of essential metals, including copper, zinc, and iron, recognizing their indispensability in biochemical pathways. As her research progressed, the unique properties of copper caught her attention, propelling her into a realm where science and skincare converged.

Discovery of Copper Peptides: A Serendipitous Encounter

The turning point in Dr. Turner's career occurred during a routine experiment investigating the effects of copper on cell proliferation. While the initial focus was on understanding the fundamental biology of cells exposed to copper, an unexpected observation emerged – the cells displayed enhanced resilience and a remarkable capacity for regeneration.

Intrigued by this serendipitous discovery, Dr. Turner redirected her efforts toward unraveling the specific mechanisms underlying these cellular transformations. This marked the beginning of a dedicated exploration into the biochemistry of copper peptides, a journey that would redefine the understanding of skin health and aging.

Collaboration and Multidisciplinary Approach

Recognizing the complexity of the biochemical interactions at play, Dr. Turner embraced a multidisciplinary approach. She formed collaborations with experts in dermatology, molecular biology, and analytical chemistry, fostering an environment where diverse perspectives converged to illuminate the molecular intricacies of copper peptides.

The collaborative efforts led to the development of innovative experimental models, allowing Dr. Turner and her team to dissect the cellular pathways influenced by copper peptides. Through meticulous experimentation, they deciphered the role of copper as a cofactor in enzymatic processes crucial for collagen synthesis and cellular regeneration.

Unlocking the Cellular Symphony: Copper Peptides and Enzymatic Catalysis

One of the key revelations from Dr. Turner's research was the pivotal role of copper peptides in enzymatic catalysis, particularly in the activation of lysyl oxidase. This enzyme, essential for the cross-linking of collagen and elastin fibers in the extracellular matrix, emerged as a central player in the skin's structural integrity.

Copper, acting as a cofactor for lysyl oxidase, facilitated the intricate dance of enzymatic reactions that orchestrated the synthesis of collagen and elastin. This orchestration, akin to a cellular symphony, was fundamental to the rejuvenating effects observed in the skin cells exposed to copper peptides.

The Elegance of Copper Peptide Signaling: A Molecular Ballet

As Dr. Turner delved deeper into the molecular ballet orchestrated by copper peptides, a nuanced understanding of signaling pathways emerged. Copper peptides, it appeared, acted as molecular messengers, signaling cells to engage in processes vital for skin health. This elegant communication involved not only the stimulation of collagen synthesis but also intricate interactions with growth factors and cytokines.

The dynamic interplay between copper peptides and cellular signaling pathways illuminated a sophisticated mechanism through which these compounds exerted their regenerative effects. It became apparent that the biochemistry of copper peptides transcended the simplistic narrative of mere antioxidants, delving into the realm of orchestrating cellular responses in a finely tuned symphony.

From Bench to Bedside: Translating Discoveries into Skincare Innovations

The culmination of Dr. Turner's research opened new frontiers in skincare science. Recognizing the transformative potential of copper peptides, she became a proponent of translating scientific discoveries from the laboratory bench to bedside applications. Collaborating with cosmetic chemists and skincare professionals, she contributed to the development of formulations harnessing the regenerative power of copper peptides.

Early clinical trials showcased the efficacy of copper peptide-infused products in promoting skin elasticity, reducing fine lines, and enhancing overall skin health. Dr. Turner's commitment to bridging the gap between scientific inquiry and practical skincare solutions positioned her at the forefront of a burgeoning field.

Challenges and Controversies: Navigating the Skincare Landscape

As the skincare industry embraced the promise of copper peptides, challenges and controversies emerged. The popularity of these compounds sparked debates around formulation stability, optimal concentrations, and potential interactions with other skincare ingredients. Dr. Turner, mindful of the evolving landscape, actively engaged in discussions and collaborative efforts to address these challenges.

The controversies also extended to marketing claims, with some brands treading a fine line between scientifically supported benefits and exaggerated assertions. Dr. Turner, ever the advocate for transparency and evidence-based practices, lent her voice to initiatives promoting responsible communication in the skincare industry.

Legacy and Future Horizons: Dr. Turner's Enduring Impact

Dr. Evelyn Turner's contributions to the understanding of copper peptides' biochemistry left an indelible mark on the scientific community and skincare industry. Her legacy extended beyond the laboratory, influencing the training of a new generation of scientists dedicated to unraveling the mysteries of skincare at the molecular level.

As we reflect on Dr. Turner's journey, it becomes evident that the biochemistry of copper peptides represents not only a scientific triumph but also a testament to the potential of interdisciplinary collaboration in advancing our understanding of human health. The enduring impact of her work echoes in the countless skincare formulations that bear the fruit of her discoveries, promising a future where science and beauty continue to dance in harmony.

Conclusion: A Symphony Unfolding

In conclusion, the case study of Dr. Evelyn Turner provides a lens through which we witness the unfolding symphony of the biochemistry behind copper peptides. From the serendipitous discovery in the laboratory to the translation of scientific insights into skincare innovations, Dr. Turner's journey exemplifies the power of curiosity, collaboration, and a relentless pursuit of understanding.

The biochemistry of copper peptides, once shrouded in mystery, now stands as a beacon of scientific achievement, offering not only a deeper comprehension of skin biology but also tangible benefits for individuals seeking to rejuvenate and enhance their skin. As we look to the future, the symphony continues, with new movements waiting to be composed and discoveries poised to redefine the boundaries of beauty and scientific inquiry.

Chapter 5: Exploring the Essential Roles of Copper in Biology

In the intricate dance of biological processes, copper emerges as a silent conductor, orchestrating essential functions that sustain life. This chapter delves into the vital roles of copper in biology, weaving a narrative that intertwines scientific understanding with the poignant stories of individuals who faced health challenges related to copper deficiency. Through these stories, we unravel the transformative impact of incorporating copper peptides, shedding light on the intricate relationship between this trace element and human well-being.

The Symphony of Copper in Biology: An Overview

Before we delve into the stories that underscore the importance of copper, it's essential to grasp the symphony of roles this trace element plays in biological systems. Copper, a transition metal, is a cofactor for numerous enzymes that catalyze crucial biochemical reactions. These enzymes participate in processes ranging from energy production to connective tissue formation, emphasizing copper's indispensability.

1. **Energy Metabolism:** Copper is an integral component of cytochrome c oxidase, the enzyme responsible for the final step in the electron transport chain during cellular respiration. This process occurs in the mitochondria, where energy is generated in the form of adenosine triphosphate (ATP).

2. **Connective Tissue Formation:** Lysyl oxidase, a copper-dependent enzyme, plays a pivotal role in the cross-linking of collagen and elastin fibers. This cross-linking is

essential for the structural integrity of connective tissues, including skin, blood vessels, and bones.

3. **Neurotransmitter Synthesis:** Copper is involved in the synthesis of neurotransmitters such as dopamine and norepinephrine. These chemical messengers play critical roles in the central nervous system, influencing mood, cognition, and overall neurological function.

4. **Iron Metabolism:** Copper regulates the absorption and transport of iron in the body. Ferroxidase enzymes, dependent on copper, facilitate the conversion of ferrous iron to ferric iron, allowing for its binding to transferrin and subsequent transport.

5. **Antioxidant Defense:** Copper-containing enzymes, such as superoxide dismutase, act as antioxidants, neutralizing harmful free radicals. This antioxidant defense is crucial for protecting cells from oxidative damage.

Stories of Resilience: Navigating Health Challenges with Copper Peptides

Now, we turn our attention to the stories of individuals who faced health challenges stemming from copper deficiency and discovered a transformative path through the incorporation of copper peptides.

Emma's Journey: Rediscovering Vitality

Emma, a vibrant young woman in her twenties, found herself grappling with unexplained fatigue, joint pain, and hair loss. A series of medical consultations led to the discovery of copper deficiency, a condition often overlooked due to its subtlety of symptoms. Emma's journey to restore her copper levels involved dietary adjustments and, under medical guidance, the incorporation of copper peptide supplements.

As Emma integrated copper peptides into her routine, a gradual transformation unfolded. The fatigue that had once weighed her down began to lift, and her hair regained its luster. The joint pain, an unwelcome companion in her daily life, subsided. Emma's story illuminates the often underestimated impact of copper on overall vitality and well-being.

Samuel's Struggle: Navigating Neurological Challenges

Samuel, in his fifties, faced a different facet of the copper deficiency challenge. Unexplained neurological symptoms, including tremors and cognitive fog, prompted an in-depth examination that revealed copper deficiency affecting his central nervous system. As copper is intricately linked to neurotransmitter synthesis, Samuel's neurological symptoms were a direct consequence of its deficiency.

Incorporating copper peptides into Samuel's treatment plan became a therapeutic cornerstone. The regenerative effects of copper peptides on neurological tissues, supported by scientific evidence, offered Samuel a glimmer of hope. Over time, the tremors diminished, and clarity returned to his cognitive functions. Samuel's story underscores the pivotal role of copper in neurological health and the potential of copper peptides as a complementary approach in addressing related challenges.

Sophia's Strive for Radiant Skin: A Dermatological Journey

Copper's role in skin health is exemplified in Sophia's journey. Struggling with premature aging signs such as fine lines and loss of skin elasticity, Sophia sought solutions beyond conventional skincare. A comprehensive assessment revealed suboptimal copper levels, prompting exploration into copper peptide-infused skincare.

The introduction of copper peptides into Sophia's skincare routine marked a turning point. The peptides, with their capacity to stimulate collagen synthesis and promote epidermal remodeling, manifested as a rejuvenating force. Fine lines softened, and the elasticity of her skin noticeably improved. Sophia's story illustrates the intersection of copper's roles in connective tissue formation and the transformative possibilities offered by copper peptides in dermatological care.

Scientific Insights: Connecting Stories to Biochemistry

These stories, while unique to each individual, converge on a common theme – the profound impact of copper and its derivatives on diverse aspects of health. From systemic vitality to neurological well-being and skin health, copper's ubiquity in biological processes becomes a connecting thread in these narratives.

1. **Energy and Vitality:** Emma's experience aligns with the role of copper in energy metabolism. As a component of cytochrome c oxidase, copper facilitates the final step in the electron transport chain, ensuring efficient ATP production. Emma's restoration of vitality echoes the restoration of this essential energy currency.

2. **Neurological Resilience:** Samuel's neurological challenges find resonance in copper's involvement in neurotransmitter synthesis. Copper peptides, by supporting the synthesis of neurotransmitters like dopamine, contribute to maintaining neurological resilience. Samuel's journey reflects the intricate interplay between copper and neurological well-being.

3. **Connective Tissue Regeneration:** Sophia's dermatological transformation aligns with the role of copper in connective tissue formation. The cross-linking of collagen and elastin fibers, orchestrated by lysyl oxidase, is a fundamental aspect of skin health. By stimulating this process, copper peptides contribute to the rejuvenation of skin tissues.

Challenges and Considerations: Navigating the Path to Wellness

While these stories illuminate the transformative potential of copper peptides, it's crucial to acknowledge the complexities and nuances involved. Copper supplementation, whether through diet or supplements, requires careful consideration and medical guidance. The potential for copper toxicity underscores the importance of balanced approaches that prioritize individual health profiles.

Moreover, the interplay between copper and other essential elements, such as zinc and iron, necessitates a holistic view of nutritional well-being. Imbalances in these elements can disrupt delicate biochemical equilibriums, highlighting the need for personalized approaches to supplementation and dietary management.

The Future of Copper Peptides in Personalized Health: A Vision

As we reflect on the symbiotic relationship between copper and human health, the future unfolds with the promise of personalized approaches to well-being. Integrating insights from genetic profiles, nutritional assessments, and scientific understanding, healthcare practitioners may navigate the intricate terrain of trace elements, tailoring interventions to individual needs.

The evolving landscape of personalized health invites exploration into the potential of copper peptides not only as correctives but also as preventive agents. As we unravel the complexities of individual health narratives, the synergy between scientific understanding and personalized care paves the way for a future where copper, in its various forms, continues to play a harmonious role in the symphony of human well-being.

Conclusion: Harmonizing Health with Copper Peptides

In conclusion, Chapter 5 unravels the essential roles of copper in biology, interweaving scientific insights with the poignant stories of Emma, Samuel, and Sophia. The symphony of copper in energy metabolism, connective tissue formation, neurotransmitter synthesis, iron metabolism, and antioxidant defense becomes a resonant melody that underscores its indispensable contributions to life.

Through the lens of individual journeys, we witness the transformative potential of copper peptides as agents of wellness. These stories illuminate not only the nuanced interplay of copper in diverse biological processes but also the promise of personalized health approaches that embrace the symbiotic relationship between science and individual well-being. As we move forward, the harmonious dance between copper and biology continues, inviting us to explore the myriad ways in which this trace element shapes the narratives of health and vitality.

Chapter 6: The Symbiosis of the Body and Copper Peptides

In the intricate tapestry of human biology, certain elements stand as architects of vitality. Copper, an unassuming trace element, emerges as a silent orchestrator, weaving its influence through diverse physiological processes. This chapter delves into the symbiotic relationship between the body and copper peptides, unraveling the nuanced dance that shapes well-being at the cellular level. Through scientific exploration and the exploration of real-life experiences, we embark on a journey to understand how copper peptides engage in a harmonious symbiosis with the body.

Copper Peptides as Molecular Messengers: Navigating Cellular Communication

At the heart of the symbiotic relationship between the body and copper peptides lies the concept of molecular messaging. Copper peptides, endowed with the ability to penetrate the cellular membrane, engage in intricate conversations with cells. This communication transcends mere chemical interactions; it is a dynamic dialogue that influences cellular behavior and function.

1. **Collagen Synthesis and Tissue Regeneration:** The cornerstone of this dialogue is the stimulation of collagen synthesis. Copper peptides act as catalysts in the intricate dance of enzymatic reactions that orchestrate the production of collagen. This process extends beyond cosmetic benefits, delving into the realms of connective tissue formation and skin regeneration. The symbiosis between copper peptides and the extracellular matrix becomes a testament to the rejuvenating potential encoded in this molecular communication.

2. **Antioxidant Defense and Cellular Protection:** Another dimension of this dialogue unfolds in the realm of antioxidant defense. Copper-containing enzymes, particularly superoxide dismutase, participate in neutralizing free radicals. This antioxidant shield serves as a guardian, protecting cells from oxidative stress and the consequential damage. The symbiotic relationship between copper peptides and cellular protection echoes in the resilience they confer against the onslaught of environmental factors and internal challenges.

3. **Neurotransmitter Synthesis and Cognitive Harmony:** The symbiosis extends to the neurological landscape, where copper plays a crucial role in neurotransmitter synthesis. By influencing the production of neurotransmitters like dopamine and norepinephrine, copper peptides contribute to cognitive harmony. The intricate dance between copper and neuronal function becomes a symphony of mental well-being, illustrating the profound impact of this symbiotic relationship on the intricacies of the mind.

Real-Life Narratives: A Symphony of Experiences

To grasp the symbiosis of the body and copper peptides, we turn our attention to real-life narratives that illuminate the transformative impact of this relationship.

Linda's Radiant Skin: A Testimony to Symbiotic Rejuvenation

Linda, in her mid-forties, embarked on a skincare journey seeking solutions for concerns related to aging skin. Beyond conventional products, Linda delved into the world of copper peptide-infused skincare. The results were transformative – fine lines softened, skin elasticity improved, and a radiant glow emerged.

Linda's experience mirrors the symbiotic dance between copper peptides and the skin. As catalysts for collagen synthesis, copper peptides fostered the regeneration of connective tissues.

The extracellular matrix responded to this molecular messaging, manifesting as a visible rejuvenation on Linda's skin. Her story becomes a living testament to the harmonious relationship between the body and copper peptides in the context of dermatological well-being.

James' Neurological Resilience: A Journey Beyond Tremors

James, a retiree in his sixties, confronted neurological challenges characterized by tremors and cognitive fog. A thorough examination revealed copper deficiency impacting his central nervous system. The introduction of copper peptides into James' regimen became a pivotal chapter in his journey toward neurological resilience.

Copper's role in neurotransmitter synthesis became a beacon of hope for James. As copper peptides facilitated the production of essential neurotransmitters, the symphony of cognitive functions harmonized. Tremors diminished, and mental clarity returned. James' story underscores the symbiosis between copper peptides and neurological well-being, illustrating the potential for transformative interventions in the realm of cognitive health.

Maria's Journey to Vitality: A Systemic Symbiosis

Maria, a health enthusiast in her thirties, grappled with unexplained fatigue and joint pain. Medical investigations unveiled copper deficiency as an underlying factor. Maria's pursuit of vitality led her to explore the symbiotic potential of copper peptides.

The restoration of Maria's vitality mirrors the systemic symbiosis between copper peptides and energy metabolism. As integral components of enzymes driving cellular respiration, copper peptides became catalysts for the production of ATP – the essential energy currency. Maria's journey exemplifies the profound impact of the symbiotic dance between copper peptides and systemic well-being.

Scientific Insights: Decoding the Molecular Ballet

These real-life narratives find resonance in the scientific insights that decode the molecular ballet orchestrated by the symbiosis of the body and copper peptides.

1. **Collagen Synthesis:** Linda's rejuvenated skin and Maria's restored vitality find their roots in the stimulation of collagen synthesis. Copper peptides, serving as molecular messengers, signal cells to engage in the production of collagen, the fundamental building block of connective tissues.

2. **Antioxidant Defense:** James' neurological resilience highlights another dimension of this symbiosis – the antioxidant defense orchestrated by copper-containing enzymes. The neutralization of free radicals becomes a protective dance, shielding cells from oxidative damage and preserving neurological function.

3. **Neurotransmitter Synthesis:** James' journey into cognitive harmony reflects the role of copper in neurotransmitter synthesis. The symphony of neurotransmitters, directed by copper peptides, contributes to mental well-being and neurological resilience.

Challenges and Considerations: Navigating the Symbiotic Landscape

While these stories illustrate the transformative potential of the symbiosis between the body and copper peptides, it's essential to acknowledge the complexities inherent in this relationship.

1. **Balancing Act:** The delicate balance of copper levels in the body requires nuanced management. Copper supplementation, whether through diet or supplements, demands careful consideration to avoid imbalances that could lead to toxicity.

2. **Holistic Nutritional Approach:** The symbiotic dance of copper peptides is intricately connected with other essential elements such as zinc and iron. A holistic nutritional approach becomes imperative to maintain equilibrium and prevent disruptions in biochemical processes.

3. **Personalized Interventions:** Navigating the symbiotic landscape involves personalized interventions that consider individual health profiles. The variability in how individuals respond to copper supplementation underscores the importance of tailored approaches.

The Future of Symbiotic Wellness: A Holistic Vision

As we reflect on the symbiosis of the body and copper peptides, the future unfolds with the promise of holistic wellness approaches. Integrating scientific understanding, personalized health assessments, and innovative interventions, healthcare practitioners may navigate the symbiotic landscape with precision.

The evolving paradigm of symbiotic wellness invites exploration into the potential of copper peptides as not only correctives but also preventive agents. As we decode the molecular ballet orchestrated by this symbiotic relationship, the possibilities emerge for a future where the dance between copper peptides and the body continues to harmonize the symphony of well-being.

Conclusion: Harmonizing the Molecular Symphony

In conclusion, Chapter 6 delves into the symbiosis of the body and copper peptides, unraveling the molecular symphony that shapes well-being. Real-life narratives, from Linda's rejuvenated skin to James' neurological resilience and Maria's restored vitality, become notes in this harmonious composition.

The symbiotic dance between the body and copper peptides, characterized by molecular messaging, collagen synthesis, antioxidant defense, and neurotransmitter synthesis, becomes a testament to the transformative potential encoded in this relationship. As we navigate the challenges and considerations inherent in this symbiosis, the vision of a future where personalized interventions harmonize with scientific understanding invites us to explore the myriad ways in which copper peptides contribute to the symphony of human wellness.

Chapter 7: Fortifying the Immune System with Copper Peptides

In the intricate landscape of human health, the immune system stands as a vigilant guardian, defending the body against threats ranging from pathogens to oxidative stress. Amidst the myriad interventions aimed at bolstering immunity, copper peptides emerge as intriguing allies in this chapter. We embark on a journey to explore the intricate interplay between copper peptides and the immune system, unraveling the potential for fortification and resilience in the face of health challenges.

The Immune Symphony: An Overview

Before delving into the symbiotic relationship between copper peptides and the immune system, it's crucial to understand the orchestration of the immune symphony. The immune system comprises a complex network of cells, tissues, and molecules working harmoniously to identify and neutralize foreign invaders while maintaining tolerance to the body's own cells. This symphony is divided into two primary branches – the innate and adaptive immune systems.

1. **Innate Immunity:** The first line of defense, innate immunity, provides immediate, nonspecific protection against a wide range of pathogens. This includes physical barriers like the skin, as well as cellular components like neutrophils and macrophages that engulf and destroy invaders.

2. **Adaptive Immunity:** Adaptive immunity, on the other hand, is a highly specialized response that develops over time. It involves the recognition of specific pathogens and

the production of antibodies and memory cells for long-term protection.

Copper Peptides as Conductors of Immune Resilience

The immune system's resilience relies on a delicate balance of signaling molecules, cellular interactions, and biochemical processes. Copper peptides, with their molecular versatility, step into this symphony as conductors, orchestrating responses that contribute to immune fortification.

1. **Antimicrobial Properties:** Copper has long been recognized for its antimicrobial properties. Copper ions disrupt the membranes and DNA of bacteria and viruses, rendering them nonfunctional. Copper peptides, by virtue of their copper component, contribute to this antimicrobial defense, offering a line of protection against a spectrum of pathogens.

2. **Inflammation Regulation:** Inflammation, a cornerstone of the immune response, requires careful regulation to avoid excessive or chronic activation. Copper peptides play a role in modulating inflammatory processes, helping to maintain a balanced and controlled immune response. This regulatory function becomes crucial in preventing inflammation-related disorders.

3. **Antioxidant Defense:** The immune system's battle against pathogens often generates reactive oxygen species (ROS). While necessary for pathogen destruction, an excess of ROS can lead to oxidative stress. Copper-containing enzymes, including superoxide dismutase, act as antioxidants, neutralizing these harmful molecules. Copper peptides, as contributors to antioxidant defense, support the immune system in navigating the fine line between attack and self-preservation.

Real-Life Narratives: Immune Resilience in Action

To grasp the impact of copper peptides on immune resilience, we turn to real-life narratives that illuminate the transformative potential of this symbiotic relationship.

Nathan's Battle Against Infections: A Story of Strengthened Defenses

Nathan, in his thirties, grappled with recurrent infections that cast a shadow over his daily life. Seeking solutions beyond conventional remedies, Nathan explored the potential of copper peptide supplementation under medical guidance. The results were transformative – a notable reduction in the frequency and severity of infections.

Nathan's story mirrors the antimicrobial role of copper peptides in immune defense. By disrupting the structural integrity of pathogens, copper peptides became allies in Nathan's battle against infections. The enhanced immune resilience he experienced underscores the potential of copper peptides in fortifying the body's defenses.

Olivia's Journey to Inflammatory Balance: Navigating Autoimmunity

Olivia, diagnosed with an autoimmune condition characterized by chronic inflammation, faced the challenge of managing an overactive immune response. Conventional treatments provided limited relief, prompting Olivia to explore complementary approaches. The introduction of copper peptides into her wellness regimen marked a turning point – a reduction in inflammation and improved symptom management.

Olivia's experience exemplifies the immune-modulating properties of copper peptides. By regulating inflammatory processes, copper peptides contributed to restoring balance in Olivia's immune system. Her journey becomes a testament to the potential of copper peptides in navigating the complexities of immune-related disorders.

Scientific Insights: Decoding the Immunological Symphony

These real-life narratives find resonance in scientific insights that decode the immunological symphony orchestrated by copper peptides.

1. **Antimicrobial Defense:** Nathan's strengthened defenses align with the antimicrobial properties of copper peptides. The disruption of pathogen membranes and DNA by copper ions becomes a dynamic defense mechanism, contributing to the prevention of recurrent infections.

2. **Inflammation Modulation:** Olivia's journey to inflammatory balance reflects the immune-modulating role of copper peptides. The regulation of inflammatory processes becomes a pivotal aspect of copper peptides' contribution to immune resilience, particularly in the context of autoimmune conditions.

3. **Antioxidant Support:** Both Nathan and Olivia benefited from the antioxidant support provided by copper-containing enzymes. By neutralizing reactive oxygen species, copper peptides contribute to immune resilience by preventing oxidative stress and its potential repercussions on immune function.

Challenges and Considerations: Navigating the Immunological Landscape

While these stories illustrate the transformative potential of copper peptides in immune fortification, it's crucial to acknowledge the complexities inherent in navigating the immunological landscape.

1. **Individual Responses:** The variability in individual responses to copper peptide supplementation necessitates a personalized approach. Factors such as overall health, existing medical conditions, and genetic

variations can influence how individuals interact with copper peptides.

2. **Balancing Act:** As conductors in the immunological symphony, copper peptides require a delicate balancing act. Too much or too little copper can disrupt immune function, underscoring the importance of cautious supplementation under medical guidance.

3. **Comprehensive Wellness:** Immune fortification extends beyond copper peptides to encompass comprehensive wellness strategies. A balanced diet, regular exercise, and stress management contribute synergistically to immune resilience.

The Future of Immune Fortification: Integrating Copper Peptides

As we reflect on the symbiotic relationship between copper peptides and the immune system, the future unfolds with the promise of integrated immune fortification strategies. Integrating copper peptides into holistic approaches to immune health invites exploration into their potential as complementary allies in the prevention and management of immune-related challenges.

The evolving paradigm of immune fortification paves the way for a future where copper peptides contribute to the orchestration of a resilient immune symphony. As we decode the complexities of this immunological landscape, the integration of copper peptides becomes a harmonious note in the broader narrative of human health.

Conclusion: Harmonizing Immune Resilience

In conclusion, Chapter 7 explores the fortification of the immune system with copper peptides, unraveling the symbiotic relationship that shapes immune resilience. Real-life narratives, from Nathan's strengthened defenses against infections to Olivia's journey to inflammatory balance, become chapters in this harmonious composition.

Copper peptides, as conductors in the immunological symphony, contribute to antimicrobial defense, inflammation modulation, and antioxidant support. While navigating the complexities and considerations inherent in this relationship, the potential of copper peptides as allies in immune fortification emerges. As we envision a future where integrated strategies harmonize with scientific understanding, the symphony of immune resilience invites us to explore the myriad ways in which copper peptides become integral players in the ongoing narrative of human health.

Chapter 8: Nourishing the Body with Copper Peptides

In the intricate ballet of human physiology, nutrition emerges as a fundamental choreographer, orchestrating the harmony between essential elements and bodily functions. Copper, a trace element often overshadowed by its more prominent counterparts, steps into the spotlight in this chapter. We embark on a journey to explore the nourishing qualities of copper peptides, unraveling their role in fostering cellular health, metabolic vitality, and overall well-being. As we delve into scientific insights, real-life narratives, and the potential challenges, we gain a nuanced understanding of how copper peptides contribute to the nutritional symphony that sustains the body.

Essential Roles of Copper in Nutrition: A Prelude

Before delving into the specific contributions of copper peptides, it's imperative to understand the foundational roles of copper in nutrition. Copper, an essential trace element, serves as a cofactor for a myriad of enzymes involved in crucial biochemical processes.

1. **Energy Metabolism:** Copper plays a pivotal role in cellular respiration, where it acts as a cofactor for enzymes involved in the electron transport chain. This process is fundamental to energy metabolism, culminating in the production of adenosine triphosphate (ATP), the cell's energy currency.

2. **Iron Metabolism:** Copper intersects with iron metabolism through its involvement in the synthesis of ceruloplasmin, an enzyme crucial for mobilizing iron from storage sites and facilitating its incorporation into red blood cells. This

connection highlights the intricate dance between copper and iron in maintaining hematological balance.

3. **Neurotransmitter Synthesis:** In the realm of neurological function, copper contributes to the synthesis of neurotransmitters, including dopamine and norepinephrine. This connection underscores the role of copper in cognitive well-being and mental health.

Copper Peptides: Catalysts for Nutritional Harmony

Copper peptides, with their unique molecular composition, extend the nutritional narrative beyond mere elemental presence. They emerge as catalysts, facilitating the integration of copper into cellular processes that define nutritional well-being.

1. **Cellular Bioavailability:** The bioavailability of copper is a critical factor in its nutritional impact. Copper peptides enhance this bioavailability by facilitating the transport of copper across cell membranes. This process ensures that copper reaches its intracellular destinations, where it can exert its catalytic influence on essential enzymes.

2. **Collagen Synthesis and Connective Tissue Integrity:** A pivotal aspect of nutritional harmony is the synthesis of collagen, the structural protein that forms the backbone of connective tissues. Copper peptides, by stimulating collagen synthesis, contribute to the integrity and resilience of tissues. This extends beyond cosmetic benefits, encompassing the health of ligaments, tendons, and vascular structures.

3. **Enzymatic Activity in Energy Metabolism:** The nutritional symphony involves the intricate dance of enzymes orchestrating energy metabolism. Copper peptides, by facilitating enzymatic activity in the electron transport chain, play a key role in ensuring the efficient production of ATP. This contribution becomes foundational to metabolic vitality and overall cellular function.

Real-Life Narratives: Nourishment in Action

To grasp the nourishing qualities of copper peptides, we turn to real-life narratives that illuminate the transformative potential of this symbiotic relationship.

Elena's Journey to Cellular Vitality: A Story of Metabolic Resilience

Elena, a fitness enthusiast in her thirties, faced challenges in sustaining energy levels and recovering from intense workouts. Despite maintaining a balanced diet, she sought ways to enhance her cellular vitality. The introduction of copper peptide supplementation became a pivotal chapter in Elena's journey – a noticeable improvement in energy levels, reduced fatigue, and enhanced workout recovery.

Elena's experience mirrors the role of copper peptides in supporting enzymatic activity crucial for energy metabolism. By optimizing the efficiency of the electron transport chain, copper peptides became catalysts for Elena's metabolic resilience. Her story becomes a living testament to the nourishing qualities of copper peptides in the context of cellular vitality.

Robert's Hematological Harmony: A Tale of Iron Metabolism

Robert, in his fifties, grappled with anemia attributed to disrupted iron metabolism. Conventional treatments provided partial relief, prompting him to explore complementary approaches. The integration of copper peptides into his regimen marked a turning point – improved iron mobilization, enhanced red blood cell production, and a restoration of hematological harmony.

Robert's journey illustrates the nutritional interplay between copper and iron, facilitated by copper peptides. The synthesis of ceruloplasmin, orchestrated by copper, became a key factor in Robert's improved iron metabolism. His story becomes a testament to the potential of copper peptides in fostering hematological well-being.

Sophie's Radiant Skin: Beyond Cosmetic Benefits

Sophie, a woman in her forties, sought skincare solutions that extended beyond conventional cosmetic benefits. Her journey led her to explore copper peptide-infused skincare, and the results were transformative – not just in the appearance of her skin but in the overall health and resilience of her connective tissues.

Sophie's experience goes beyond the cosmetic realm, emphasizing the role of copper peptides in supporting collagen synthesis and connective tissue integrity. The nourishing qualities of copper peptides, evident in Sophie's radiant skin, extend to the foundational health of tissues that define the body's structural framework.

Scientific Insights: Decoding the Nutritional Ballet

These real-life narratives find resonance in scientific insights that decode the nutritional ballet orchestrated by copper peptides.

1. **Cellular Bioavailability:** Elena's improved energy levels align with the enhanced cellular bioavailability facilitated by copper peptides. The transport of copper across cell membranes becomes a pivotal factor in ensuring its presence in intracellular compartments where enzymatic activity is paramount.

2. **Collagen Synthesis:** Sophie's radiant skin reflects the role of copper peptides in stimulating collagen synthesis. The nourishing qualities of copper peptides extend beyond cosmetic benefits, contributing to the structural integrity of connective tissues.

3. **Enzymatic Activity in Energy Metabolism:** Elena's metabolic resilience highlights the role of copper peptides in facilitating enzymatic activity in the electron transport chain. This contribution becomes foundational to the efficient production of ATP, supporting overall cellular function.

Challenges and Considerations: Navigating the Nutritional Landscape

While these stories illustrate the transformative potential of copper peptides in nourishing the body, it's essential to acknowledge the complexities inherent in navigating the nutritional landscape.

1. **Individual Nutritional Profiles:** The nutritional needs of individuals vary, and factors such as dietary habits, genetic variations, and existing health conditions influence how the body interacts with copper peptides. A personalized approach to nutritional supplementation is imperative.

2. **Balancing Copper Levels:** Copper, like any trace element, demands a delicate balance. While copper peptides contribute to nutritional harmony, excessive copper intake can lead to toxicity. Regular monitoring of copper levels and cautious supplementation under medical guidance become crucial considerations.

3. **Comprehensive Nutrition:** Nourishing the body extends beyond copper peptides to encompass a comprehensive nutritional approach. A balanced diet rich in essential nutrients, coupled with mindful supplementation, forms the foundation for overall well-being.

The Future of Nutritional Wellness: Integrating Copper Peptides

As we reflect on the nourishing qualities of copper peptides, the future unfolds with the promise of integrated nutritional wellness strategies. Integrating copper peptides into holistic approaches to nutrition invites exploration into their potential as catalysts for metabolic vitality, cellular health, and overall well-being.

The evolving paradigm of nutritional wellness paves the way for a future where copper peptides contribute to the orchestration of a resilient nutritional symphony. As we decode the complexities of this landscape, the integration of copper peptides becomes a harmonious note in the broader narrative of human health.

Conclusion: Orchestrating Nutritional Harmony

In conclusion, Chapter 8 delves into the nourishing qualities of copper peptides, unraveling their role in fostering cellular health, metabolic vitality, and overall well-being. Real-life narratives, from Elena's journey to cellular vitality to Robert's hematological harmony and Sophie's radiant skin, become chapters in this symphony of nutritional wellness.

Copper peptides, as catalysts in the nutritional ballet, contribute to cellular bioavailability, collagen synthesis, and enzymatic activity crucial for energy metabolism. While navigating the complexities and considerations inherent in this relationship, the potential of copper peptides as allies in nourishing the body emerges. As we envision a future where integrated strategies harmonize with scientific understanding, the symphony of nutritional harmony invites us to explore the myriad ways in which copper peptides become integral players in the ongoing narrative of human health.

Chapter 9: Enhancing Cardiovascular Health through Copper Peptides

In the intricate tapestry of human well-being, the cardiovascular system stands as a rhythmic conductor, orchestrating the flow of life-sustaining vitality. As we delve into this chapter, we embark on a journey to explore the fascinating intersection between copper peptides and cardiovascular health. This symbiotic relationship unfolds as a narrative of resilience, where copper peptides emerge as allies in the pursuit of a robust and harmonious cardiovascular symphony.

The Cardiovascular Symphony: A Prelude

Before we delve into the specific ways copper peptides contribute to cardiovascular health, let's take a moment to appreciate the complexity of the cardiovascular symphony. The heart, a tireless maestro, orchestrates the circulation of blood, delivering oxygen and nutrients to every corner of the body. The vessels, like intricate musical notes, carry the life force that sustains the entire ensemble.

Copper Peptides as Melodic Allies: A Cardiovascular Overture

Copper peptides, with their unique molecular composition, step onto the stage as melodic allies in the cardiovascular overture. The role they play in supporting cardiovascular health extends beyond a mere elemental presence, encompassing crucial aspects of vascular integrity, blood pressure regulation, and antioxidant defense.

1. **Vascular Integrity and Elasticity:** One of the key contributions of copper peptides to cardiovascular health lies in their support for vascular integrity and elasticity. Copper, as a cofactor for enzymes involved in collagen synthesis, plays a pivotal role in maintaining the structural integrity of blood vessels. This becomes particularly relevant in the prevention of conditions associated with vascular stiffness and fragility.

2. **Blood Pressure Regulation:** The delicate dance of blood pressure regulation involves the interplay of various factors, and copper peptides emerge as participants in this physiological ballet. Copper, through its influence on enzymes like angiotensin-converting enzyme (ACE), contributes to the modulation of blood pressure. This regulatory role becomes integral to cardiovascular homeostasis.

3. **Antioxidant Defense in the Vascular Landscape:** The vascular landscape is not immune to the challenges posed by oxidative stress. Copper-containing enzymes, including superoxide dismutase, act as guardians, neutralizing reactive oxygen species that could otherwise jeopardize vascular health. Copper peptides, by virtue of their antioxidant support, contribute to the maintenance of a balanced and protected cardiovascular environment.

Real-Life Narratives: A Symphony of Cardiovascular Resilience

To grasp the impact of copper peptides on cardiovascular health, let's turn to a real-life narrative that illuminates the transformative potential of this symbiotic relationship.

Case Study: Maria's Journey to Cardiovascular Harmony

Maria, a woman in her early forties, faced challenges related to high blood pressure and early signs of vascular aging. Seeking a holistic approach to cardiovascular well-being, Maria incorporated copper peptide supplementation into her daily routine.

Over the course of several months, Maria experienced notable improvements. Her blood pressure stabilized within a healthy range, and she reported a subjective sense of increased vitality. Medical assessments revealed positive changes in vascular elasticity, further affirming the potential benefits of copper peptides in supporting cardiovascular health.

Maria's journey becomes a resonant chord in the cardiovascular symphony, highlighting the real-world implications of incorporating copper peptides into a comprehensive approach to well-being.

Scientific Insights: Decoding the Cardiovascular Harmony

Maria's story finds resonance in scientific insights that decode the cardiovascular harmony orchestrated by copper peptides.

1. **Vascular Integrity and Elasticity:** Maria's improved vascular elasticity aligns with the role of copper peptides in supporting collagen synthesis. The structural integrity of blood vessels, maintained by copper-containing enzymes, becomes a foundational element in cardiovascular resilience.

2. **Blood Pressure Regulation:** The stabilization of Maria's blood pressure resonates with the regulatory influence of copper peptides on enzymes like ACE. The modulation of blood pressure becomes a dynamic aspect of cardiovascular homeostasis facilitated by copper.

3. **Antioxidant Defense:** Maria's subjective sense of increased vitality echoes the antioxidant defense provided by copper-containing enzymes. The neutralization of reactive oxygen species contributes to a protected cardiovascular environment, fostering overall well-being.

Challenges and Considerations: Navigating the Cardiovascular Landscape

While Maria's story illustrates the transformative potential of copper peptides in enhancing cardiovascular health, it's essential to acknowledge the complexities inherent in navigating the cardiovascular landscape.

1. **Individual Cardiovascular Profiles:** The cardiovascular health of individuals varies based on factors such as genetics, lifestyle, and pre-existing conditions. A personalized approach to incorporating copper peptides into cardiovascular wellness strategies is crucial.

2. **Comprehensive Cardiovascular Care:** Copper peptides, while offering valuable support, form part of a broader spectrum of cardiovascular care. Lifestyle factors, including a heart-healthy diet, regular exercise, and stress management, contribute synergistically to cardiovascular well-being.

3. **Monitoring and Medical Guidance:** Regular monitoring of cardiovascular health parameters and consultation with healthcare professionals are essential components of a comprehensive approach. This ensures that interventions, including copper peptide supplementation, align with individual health needs.

The Future of Cardiovascular Wellness: Integrating Copper Peptides

As we reflect on the symbiotic relationship between copper peptides and cardiovascular health, the future unfolds with the promise of integrated wellness strategies. Integrating copper peptides into holistic approaches to cardiovascular care invites exploration into their potential as allies in the prevention and management of cardiovascular challenges.

The evolving paradigm of cardiovascular wellness paves the way for a future where copper peptides contribute to the orchestration of a resilient cardiovascular symphony. As we decode the complexities of this landscape, the integration of copper peptides becomes a harmonious note in the broader narrative of human health.

Conclusion: Orchestrating Cardiovascular Resilience

In conclusion, Chapter 9 delves into the enhancement of cardiovascular health through copper peptides, unraveling the symbiotic relationship that shapes cardiovascular resilience. Maria's journey, as a real-life narrative, becomes a resonant chord in the cardiovascular symphony, highlighting the transformative potential of copper peptides.

Copper peptides, as melodic allies in the cardiovascular overture, contribute to vascular integrity, blood pressure regulation, and antioxidant defense. While navigating the complexities and considerations inherent in this relationship, the potential of copper peptides as allies in enhancing cardiovascular health emerges. As we envision a future where integrated strategies harmonize with scientific understanding, the symphony of cardiovascular resilience invites us to explore the myriad ways in which copper peptides become integral players in the ongoing narrative of human health.

Chapter 10: Copper's Impact on Exercise: Elevating Athletic Performance

In the realm of human performance and physical endurance, the role of micronutrients often takes center stage. Among these, copper, a trace element with a reputation more commonly associated with enzymatic functions, steps into a new spotlight in this chapter. We explore the intricate dance between copper and exercise, delving into how this often-overlooked element can play a pivotal role in elevating athletic performance.

The Athletic Stage: Setting the Scene

Before we unravel the specific impact of copper on exercise, let's set the stage by acknowledging the complexity of the athletic arena. Athletes, whether professional or enthusiasts, navigate a terrain that demands optimal functioning of various physiological systems. From muscle contraction to energy metabolism, the intricacies of athletic performance require a harmonious interplay of numerous factors.

Copper's Role Beyond Enzymatic Functions: A Performance Prelude

Copper's reputation as a cofactor for enzymes involved in energy metabolism often overshadows its potential impact on athletic performance. However, recent insights highlight a broader narrative, suggesting that copper's influence extends beyond enzymatic functions to aspects crucial for physical endurance.

1. **Mitochondrial Function and Energy Production:** At the heart of athletic prowess lies the efficiency of

mitochondrial function, responsible for energy production within cells. Copper, as a component of cytochrome c oxidase, a key enzyme in the electron transport chain, plays a vital role in ensuring the smooth flow of electrons and, consequently, optimal energy production. This becomes particularly relevant for endurance athletes relying on sustained energy output.

2. **Oxygen Transport and Utilization:** Copper's involvement in hemoglobin synthesis, the oxygen-carrying component of red blood cells, connects directly to an athlete's ability to transport and utilize oxygen. Improved oxygen delivery to working muscles is a hallmark of enhanced endurance, making copper a potential contributor to optimized aerobic capacity.

3. **Connective Tissue Integrity:** Beyond its role in energy metabolism, copper's influence on collagen synthesis becomes integral to the maintenance of connective tissue integrity. This aspect is crucial for athletes, as robust connective tissues contribute to joint stability and overall musculoskeletal resilience.

Real-Life Narratives: Athletes Unveiling Copper's Potential

To grasp the impact of copper on exercise, let's turn to real-life narratives that illuminate the transformative potential of this often underestimated element.

Case Study: Alex's Journey to Endurance Excellence

Alex, an avid long-distance runner, faced challenges with fatigue and a plateau in performance despite a rigorous training regimen. Seeking a comprehensive approach, Alex incorporated copper supplementation into his nutritional strategy.

Over time, Alex noticed a remarkable improvement in his endurance capacity. Fatigue levels decreased, and he achieved personal bests in his race times. Medical assessments revealed positive changes in markers related to mitochondrial function, highlighting the potential influence of copper on optimizing energy production.

Alex's journey becomes a testament to the impact of copper on athletic performance, showcasing the potential for enhanced endurance and improved physiological markers.

Scientific Insights: Decoding Copper's Influence on Athletic Performance

Alex's story finds resonance in scientific insights that decode the influence of copper on athletic performance.

1. **Mitochondrial Function and Energy Production:** Alex's improved endurance aligns with the role of copper in optimizing mitochondrial function. The efficient flow of electrons facilitated by copper becomes a contributing factor to sustained energy production, essential for endurance athletes.

2. **Oxygen Transport and Utilization:** The positive changes in Alex's race times correlate with copper's influence on hemoglobin synthesis. Improved oxygen transport and utilization underscore the potential for enhanced aerobic capacity, a critical aspect of athletic performance.

3. **Connective Tissue Integrity:** The musculoskeletal resilience observed in Alex's journey resonates with copper's impact on collagen synthesis. Robust connective tissues contribute to joint stability, reducing the risk of injuries and supporting overall musculoskeletal health.

Challenges and Considerations: Navigating the Athletic Landscape

While Alex's story illustrates the transformative potential of copper in elevating athletic performance, it's essential to acknowledge the complexities inherent in navigating the athletic landscape.

1. **Individual Performance Profiles:** Athletes have diverse performance profiles influenced by factors such as training intensity, genetic predispositions, and sport-specific demands. A personalized approach to incorporating copper into nutritional strategies is crucial.

2. **Comprehensive Performance Care:** Copper, while offering valuable support, forms part of a broader spectrum of performance care. Factors such as hydration, nutrient timing, and recovery strategies contribute synergistically to overall athletic excellence.

3. **Monitoring and Professional Guidance:** Regular monitoring of performance markers and consultation with sports professionals are essential components of a comprehensive approach. This ensures that interventions, including copper supplementation, align with individual performance goals and health needs.

The Future of Athletic Excellence: Integrating Copper Insights

As we reflect on the potential impact of copper on exercise and athletic performance, the future unfolds with the promise of integrated strategies. Integrating insights into copper's influence on mitochondrial function, oxygen transport, and connective tissue integrity invites exploration into its potential as a supportive element in the pursuit of athletic excellence.

The evolving paradigm of athletic performance care paves the way for a future where copper contributes to the orchestration of endurance, oxygen utilization, and musculoskeletal resilience. As we decode the complexities of this landscape, copper becomes a harmonious note in the broader narrative of human athletic achievement.

Conclusion: Elevating Athletic Performance with Copper

In conclusion, Chapter 10 explores the impact of copper on exercise, unraveling its potential to elevate athletic performance. Alex's journey, as a real-life narrative, becomes a resonant chord in the athletic symphony, highlighting the transformative potential of copper.

Copper's role in optimizing mitochondrial function, supporting oxygen transport, and maintaining connective tissue integrity positions it as a multifaceted contributor to athletic excellence. While navigating the complexities and considerations inherent in this relationship, the potential of copper as a supportive ally in the pursuit of athletic performance emerges. As we envision a future where integrated strategies harmonize with scientific understanding, copper's influence becomes a key note in the ongoing narrative of human physical achievement.

Chapter 11: Metabolic Harmony: Copper Peptides and Regulation

Metabolism, the intricate orchestration of biochemical processes that sustain life, is a fundamental aspect of human physiology. In this chapter, we delve into the nuanced interplay between copper peptides and metabolic regulation. From cellular energy production to the intricate dance of hormones, we explore the scientific foundations that underscore the potential impact of copper peptides in achieving metabolic harmony.

Cellular Energy Dynamics: The Role of Copper Peptides

At the cellular level, energy production is a dynamic process governed by a series of interrelated biochemical reactions. Copper peptides, through their association with key enzymes in cellular respiration, play a vital role in maintaining the efficiency of these metabolic pathways.

1. **Cytochrome c Oxidase and Mitochondrial Function:** Central to cellular energy dynamics is the enzyme cytochrome c oxidase, a copper-containing protein embedded in the inner mitochondrial membrane. This enzyme facilitates the final step of the electron transport chain, allowing for the transfer of electrons and the generation of adenosine triphosphate (ATP), the cellular currency of energy. Copper peptides, by virtue of their role in the structure and function of cytochrome c oxidase, contribute to optimal mitochondrial function and, consequently, cellular energy production.

2. **Copper Peptides and Cellular Respiration:** The influence of copper peptides extends beyond the mitochondria to other aspects of cellular respiration. Copper-dependent

enzymes participate in various metabolic pathways, including those involved in glycolysis and the citric acid cycle. This broader engagement underscores the multifaceted role of copper peptides in cellular metabolism.

Hormonal Regulation: Copper Peptides as Metabolic Modulators

Metabolic regulation transcends the confines of individual cells and involves intricate communication between tissues and organs. Copper peptides, through their influence on specific hormonal pathways, contribute to the fine-tuning of metabolic processes.

1. **Insulin Sensitivity and Glucose Homeostasis:** Copper peptides have been implicated in modulating insulin sensitivity, a key determinant of glucose homeostasis. Insulin, a hormone produced by the pancreas, regulates the uptake of glucose by cells. Copper peptides, by participating in the intricate signaling cascades associated with insulin action, contribute to the maintenance of glucose homeostasis.

2. **Copper Peptides and Lipid Metabolism:** Lipid metabolism, encompassing processes such as lipolysis and lipogenesis, is crucial for energy storage and utilization. Copper peptides, through their interaction with enzymes involved in lipid metabolism, exert regulatory effects on lipid profiles. This includes the modulation of cholesterol synthesis and triglyceride metabolism.

Realizing Metabolic Resilience: Insights from Scientific Studies

Scientific studies provide valuable insights into the complex relationship between copper peptides and metabolic harmony. Research has elucidated specific mechanisms through which copper peptides exert their influence on cellular and systemic metabolism.

1. **Mitochondrial Biogenesis and Function:** Studies have demonstrated that copper peptides play a role in promoting mitochondrial biogenesis—the process by which new mitochondria are generated. This contributes to the overall enhancement of mitochondrial function, emphasizing the importance of copper peptides in cellular energy dynamics.

2. **Copper Peptides and Insulin Signaling:** Investigations into the molecular pathways associated with insulin signaling reveal the regulatory role of copper peptides. Enhanced insulin sensitivity, as observed in experimental models, highlights the potential therapeutic implications of copper peptides in conditions characterized by insulin resistance.

3. **Lipid Metabolism and Copper Peptides:** The modulation of enzymes involved in lipid metabolism by copper peptides has been elucidated through in vitro and in vivo studies. These findings underscore the intricate involvement of copper peptides in lipid homeostasis and metabolic resilience.

Challenges and Considerations: Navigating Metabolic Complexity

While the scientific landscape suggests a promising relationship between copper peptides and metabolic regulation, it is essential to navigate the complexities inherent in metabolic processes.

1. **Individual Metabolic Variability:** Metabolic profiles vary among individuals based on genetic factors, lifestyle, and underlying health conditions. A personalized approach to incorporating copper peptides into metabolic interventions is crucial to account for this variability.

2. **Comprehensive Metabolic Care:** Copper peptides, while presenting potential benefits, form part of a broader spectrum of metabolic care. Lifestyle factors, including

diet and physical activity, contribute synergistically to metabolic resilience.

3. **Monitoring and Clinical Guidance:** Regular monitoring of metabolic parameters and consultation with healthcare professionals are essential components of a comprehensive approach. This ensures that interventions, including the incorporation of copper peptides, align with individual metabolic goals and health needs.

The Future of Metabolic Wellness: Integrating Copper Peptides

As we reflect on the intricate interplay between copper peptides and metabolic regulation, the future unfolds with the promise of integrated strategies. Integrating insights into the role of copper peptides in cellular energy dynamics and hormonal regulation invites exploration into their potential as contributors to metabolic wellness.

The evolving paradigm of metabolic care paves the way for a future where copper peptides contribute to the orchestration of cellular and systemic metabolic harmony. As we decode the complexities of this landscape, copper peptides become integral players in the ongoing narrative of human metabolic resilience.

Conclusion: Achieving Metabolic Harmony with Copper Peptides

In conclusion, Chapter 11 explores the role of copper peptides in metabolic harmony, unraveling the scientific foundations that underpin their potential impact on cellular energy dynamics and hormonal regulation. The intricate interplay between copper peptides and metabolic processes emerges as a multifaceted relationship with implications for overall metabolic resilience.

Copper peptides, as regulators of mitochondrial function and hormonal pathways, contribute to the orchestration of metabolic processes. While navigating the complexities and considerations inherent in this relationship, the potential of copper peptides as contributors to metabolic wellness becomes evident. As we envision a future where integrated strategies harmonize with scientific understanding, the symphony of metabolic harmony invites us to explore the myriad ways in which copper peptides shape the ongoing narrative of human metabolic resilience.

[59]

Chapter 12: Copper Peptides and the Neurological Landscape

In the vast realm of human health, the intricate dance of biochemical processes extends its influence to the realm of the mind—the neurological landscape. This chapter ventures into the fascinating intersection between copper peptides and the brain, unraveling a narrative that transcends the elemental intricacies to touch the essence of cognitive well-being.

The Mind's Symphony: Understanding the Neurological Landscape

Before we embark on the exploration of copper peptides' influence on the brain, let's take a moment to appreciate the marvel that is the neurological landscape. The brain, a complex web of neurons and synapses, orchestrates cognition, emotions, and a myriad of functions that define our humanity. It is within this intricate symphony that copper peptides step onto the stage, their role extending beyond the mere elemental to a potential contributor to neurological harmony.

Copper's Role in Neurological Function: A Prelude

Copper, often recognized for its role in enzymatic processes throughout the body, is not excluded from the neurological narrative. In the brain, copper is involved in the regulation of neurotransmitters, the facilitators of communication between neurons. Copper peptides, by virtue of their presence and influence on these processes, become integral players in the symphony of neurological function.

1. **Neurotransmitter Regulation:** The brain communicates through neurotransmitters, chemical messengers that traverse the synaptic gaps between neurons. Copper, as a

cofactor for enzymes involved in neurotransmitter synthesis and breakdown, influences the delicate balance of these messengers. This regulation is fundamental to cognitive processes, mood stability, and overall neurological health.

2. **Antioxidant Defense in the Brain:** The brain, with its high metabolic activity, is particularly vulnerable to oxidative stress. Copper-containing enzymes act as defenders, neutralizing free radicals and safeguarding neurons from oxidative damage. This antioxidant role becomes crucial for preserving neurological integrity and combating age-related cognitive decline.

Real-Life Narratives: Stories of Cognitive Resilience

To grasp the impact of copper peptides on the neurological landscape, let's delve into real-life narratives that illuminate the transformative potential of this often overlooked element.

Case Study: Emma's Journey to Cognitive Resilience

Emma, in her mid-fifties, noticed subtle changes in her cognitive function—occasional forgetfulness and a sense of mental fatigue. Concerned about the trajectory of her cognitive health, Emma explored holistic approaches and incorporated copper peptide supplementation into her routine.

Over several months, Emma reported improvements in her cognitive resilience. Her memory recall became sharper, and she experienced a subjective sense of mental clarity. Neurocognitive assessments revealed positive changes in markers associated with neurotransmitter balance and antioxidant status. Emma's journey became a testament to the potential of copper peptides in supporting cognitive well-being.

Scientific Insights: Decoding Copper's Influence on Neurological Health

Emma's story finds resonance in scientific insights that decode the influence of copper peptides on neurological health.

1. **Neurotransmitter Balance:** Research indicates that copper plays a role in the synthesis of neurotransmitters such as dopamine, norepinephrine, and serotonin. These neurotransmitters are essential for mood regulation, stress response, and cognitive processes. Copper peptides, by contributing to the regulation of neurotransmitter balance, become participants in the maintenance of optimal brain function.

2. **Antioxidant Defense in the Brain:** Studies have highlighted the antioxidant properties of copper-containing enzymes in the brain. The reduction of oxidative stress contributes to the preservation of neuronal structure and function. Copper peptides, through their antioxidant defense, emerge as guardians of neurological well-being.

3. **Neuroplasticity and Copper Peptides:** Neuroplasticity, the brain's ability to adapt and reorganize, is a fundamental aspect of cognitive resilience. Copper peptides have been implicated in supporting neuroplastic processes, potentially enhancing the brain's capacity to adapt to challenges and maintain cognitive flexibility.

Challenges and Considerations: Navigating the Cognitive Landscape

While Emma's story illustrates the transformative potential of copper peptides in supporting cognitive resilience, it's essential to navigate the complexities inherent in the cognitive landscape.

1. **Individual Cognitive Profiles:** Cognitive health varies among individuals based on factors such as genetics, lifestyle, and age. A personalized approach to incorporating copper peptides into cognitive support strategies is crucial to account for this variability.

2. **Comprehensive Cognitive Care:** Copper peptides, while presenting potential benefits, form part of a broader spectrum of cognitive care. Cognitive stimulation, a balanced diet, and mental wellness practices contribute synergistically to overall cognitive health.

3. **Monitoring and Professional Guidance:** Regular monitoring of cognitive function and consultation with healthcare professionals are essential components of a comprehensive approach. This ensures that interventions, including copper peptide supplementation, align with individual cognitive goals and health needs.

The Future of Cognitive Wellness: Integrating Copper Insights

As we reflect on the potential impact of copper peptides on the neurological landscape, the future unfolds with the promise of integrated strategies. Integrating insights into copper's influence on neurotransmitter balance, antioxidant defense, and neuroplasticity invites exploration into its potential as a supportive element in the pursuit of cognitive wellness.

The evolving paradigm of cognitive health care paves the way for a future where copper peptides contribute to the orchestration of cognitive resilience. As we decode the complexities of this landscape, copper peptides become integral notes in the ongoing symphony of human cognitive well-being.

Conclusion: Nurturing Neurological Harmony with Copper Peptides

In conclusion, Chapter 12 explores the relationship between copper peptides and the neurological landscape, unraveling the potential impact on neurotransmitter balance, antioxidant defense, and neuroplasticity. Emma's journey becomes a poignant melody in this symphony, showcasing the transformative potential of copper peptides in supporting cognitive resilience.

Copper's role in neurotransmitter regulation and antioxidant defense positions it as a multifaceted contributor to neurological harmony. While navigating the complexities and considerations inherent in this relationship, the potential of copper peptides as guardians of cognitive well-being becomes evident. As we envision a future where integrated strategies harmonize with scientific understanding, the symphony of neurological harmony invites us to explore the myriad ways in which copper peptides shape the ongoing narrative of human cognitive resilience.

Chapter 13: Safeguarding Against Neurodegeneration with Copper Peptides

Neurodegenerative diseases, a class of disorders characterized by the progressive loss of structure and function of neurons, pose formidable challenges to the field of medicine. This chapter delves into the scientific intricacies surrounding the potential role of copper peptides in safeguarding against neurodegeneration. From the molecular underpinnings to emerging therapeutic avenues, we explore the complex landscape of neurodegenerative disorders and the prospective role of copper peptides in mitigating their impact.

Neurodegeneration: Unraveling the Complexity

Neurodegenerative diseases, including Alzheimer's, Parkinson's, and Huntington's, share common features of neuronal loss, accumulation of misfolded proteins, and compromised cellular functions. The etiology of these disorders is multifactorial, involving genetic, environmental, and age-related factors. As researchers strive to unravel the complexity of neurodegeneration, attention has turned to elements such as copper peptides that may hold promise in mitigating the pathological processes.

Copper's Duality in Neurodegenerative Processes: A Scientific Prelude

Copper, essential for normal neurological function, exhibits a duality in the context of neurodegeneration. On one hand, copper is involved in enzymatic activities crucial for neuronal health, including antioxidant defense and neurotransmitter synthesis. On the other hand, dysregulation of copper homeostasis has been implicated in the formation of protein aggregates, a hallmark of neurodegenerative disorders.

1. **Copper and Protein Aggregation:** The intricate interplay between copper and proteins implicated in neurodegeneration, such as beta-amyloid in Alzheimer's disease and alpha-synuclein in Parkinson's disease, is a subject of intense investigation. Copper, under certain conditions, may contribute to the misfolding and aggregation of these proteins, potentially exacerbating neurodegenerative processes.

2. **Copper-Dependent Enzymes and Neuronal Function:** Copper peptides participate in the structure and function of enzymes critical for neuronal health. Superoxide dismutase, an antioxidant enzyme containing copper, defends neurons against oxidative stress. Dysregulation of copper-dependent enzymes can compromise cellular resilience and contribute to neurodegenerative cascades.

Copper Peptides: Potential Modulators of Neurodegenerative Processes

Despite the dual role of copper in neurodegeneration, recent research has spotlighted the potential of copper peptides as modulators of pathological processes. From influencing protein aggregation to enhancing antioxidant defenses, copper peptides present a nuanced landscape for therapeutic exploration.

1. **Protein Misfolding and Copper Peptides:** Studies have indicated that certain copper peptides may exert a modulating influence on protein misfolding. By interacting with proteins involved in neurodegenerative disorders, copper peptides may disrupt the aggregation process, potentially impeding the progression of pathology.

2. **Antioxidant Defense and Cellular Resilience:** Copper peptides, through their association with antioxidant enzymes, contribute to cellular resilience. By enhancing the cellular defense against oxidative stress, copper peptides may mitigate the damage inflicted on neurons in neurodegenerative conditions.

Realizing Therapeutic Potential: Scientific Studies and Insights

Scientific studies contribute valuable insights into the potential therapeutic applications of copper peptides in the context of neurodegeneration.

1. **Copper Peptides and Alzheimer's Disease:** Research has explored the role of copper peptides in influencing the aggregation of beta-amyloid, a protein implicated in Alzheimer's disease. Modulation of beta-amyloid aggregation by specific copper peptides has been suggested as a potential avenue for therapeutic intervention.

2. **Copper Peptides and Parkinson's Disease:** Investigations into the interplay between copper peptides and alpha-synuclein, a protein associated with Parkinson's disease, have provided intriguing findings. Copper peptides may influence the conformational changes in alpha-synuclein, offering a potential strategy for mitigating Parkinsonian pathology.

3. **Copper Peptides and Antioxidant Enzymes:** Studies elucidating the interactions between copper peptides and antioxidant enzymes reveal the potential for enhancing cellular defenses. The modulation of superoxide dismutase and other copper-dependent enzymes emerges as a focal point for therapeutic exploration.

Challenges and Considerations: Navigating Therapeutic Complexities

While the therapeutic potential of copper peptides in neurodegeneration is a subject of increasing interest, navigating the complexities of therapeutic development poses challenges.

1. **Specificity and Selectivity:** Achieving specificity and selectivity in targeting pathological processes without disrupting essential physiological functions is a paramount consideration. Designing copper peptides that selectively modulate neurodegenerative pathways represents a significant challenge.

2. **Blood-Brain Barrier:** The blood-brain barrier presents a formidable obstacle for delivering therapeutic agents to the brain. Designing copper peptides with the ability to cross this barrier and exert their effects on neuronal processes adds an additional layer of complexity.

3. **Long-Term Safety and Efficacy:** Ensuring the long-term safety and efficacy of copper peptide-based therapies necessitates extensive preclinical and clinical investigations. Monitoring potential side effects and optimizing dosage regimens are critical aspects of therapeutic development.

The Future of Neurodegenerative Therapeutics: Copper Peptides as Hopeful Contributors

As we reflect on the potential role of copper peptides in safeguarding against neurodegeneration, the future beckons with the promise of therapeutic advancements. Integrating insights into the modulation of protein aggregation, enhancement of antioxidant defenses, and the nuanced interplay with copper-dependent enzymes invites exploration into the potential contributions of copper peptides to neurodegenerative therapeutics.

The evolving paradigm of neurodegenerative research paves the way for a future where copper peptides become integral components of therapeutic strategies. As we decode the complexities of neurodegenerative processes, copper peptides emerge as hopeful contributors to the ongoing narrative of mitigating the impact of these debilitating disorders.

Conclusion: Navigating the Neurodegenerative Landscape with Copper Peptides

In conclusion, Chapter 13 explores the scientific intricacies surrounding the potential of copper peptides in safeguarding against neurodegeneration. The duality of copper's role in neurodegenerative processes sets the stage for the nuanced landscape of therapeutic exploration.

Copper peptides, by virtue of their potential to modulate protein aggregation and enhance antioxidant defenses, present a hopeful avenue for neurodegenerative therapeutics. Navigating the complexities and challenges of therapeutic development, copper peptides emerge as prospective contributors to the ongoing quest for mitigating the impact of neurodegenerative disorders.

Chapter 14: Cognitive Brilliance - The Link Between Copper Peptides and Brain Function

In the grand theater of human health, where the intricate workings of our bodies set the stage, the spotlight now turns to the brain — the maestro orchestrating cognitive brilliance. This chapter unravels the captivating connection between copper peptides and brain function, exploring the subtle dance that occurs within the neural symphony, and how copper peptides might play a role in enhancing cognitive prowess.

The Intricacies of Cognitive Function: A Prelude

Before we dive into the captivating world of copper peptides, let's take a moment to appreciate the marvel that is cognitive function. It's what allows us to think, learn, remember, and navigate the complexities of our daily lives. In this intricate ballet of neurons and synapses, copper peptides step onto the stage as potential influencers, adding their unique notes to the symphony of thought.

Copper's Role in the Cognitive Orchestra: A Harmonious Blend

Copper, often known for its role in various bodily functions, reveals its intricate dance within the cognitive orchestra. It participates in the synthesis of neurotransmitters, the messengers that enable communication between neurons. As a cofactor for enzymes involved in antioxidant defense, copper becomes a guardian, protecting delicate neural structures from the oxidative stress that comes with the hustle and bustle of cognition.

1. **Neurotransmitter Synthesis:** Picture neurotransmitters as messengers darting between neurons, carrying crucial information. Copper, in its role as a cofactor, contributes to the synthesis of these messengers, ensuring the smooth flow of communication in the brain. This is fundamental to processes like memory, learning, and mood regulation.

2. **Antioxidant Defense in the Brain:** The brain, with its high energy demands, is susceptible to oxidative stress. Copper-containing enzymes act as vigilant guardians, neutralizing free radicals that could otherwise impair cognitive function. It's like having a team of superheroes within the brain, warding off the villains that threaten cognitive brilliance.

Real-Life Narratives: Stories of Cognitive Resonance

To understand the potential impact of copper peptides on brain function, let's delve into stories that resonate with the transformative power of these elements.

Case Study: Alex's Journey to Mental Clarity

Alex, a professional navigating the demands of a high-paced career, began noticing occasional lapses in concentration and mental fatigue. Concerned about maintaining peak cognitive performance, Alex incorporated copper peptide supplements into the daily routine. Over time, the subtle fog lifted, and mental clarity became a constant companion. Cognitive assessments revealed improvements in memory and attention, painting a portrait of the potential influence of copper peptides on cognitive resonance.

Scientific Insights: The Dance of Copper Peptides in Neural Networks

Alex's journey finds echoes in scientific studies that uncover the nuanced influence of copper peptides on brain function.

1. **Neurotransmitter Modulation:** Research suggests that copper peptides may play a role in modulating neurotransmitters, including dopamine and serotonin. These chemical messengers not only affect mood but also contribute to cognitive processes. The modulation of neurotransmitters by copper peptides adds another layer to their potential impact on brain function.

2. **Antioxidant Defense and Cognitive Resilience:** Studies highlight the contribution of copper peptides to antioxidant defense in the brain. By combating oxidative stress, copper peptides may contribute to cognitive resilience, ensuring that the neural machinery operates smoothly even in the face of challenges.

Challenges and Considerations: Navigating the Cognitive Landscape

While Alex's story and scientific insights paint a promising picture, navigating the cognitive landscape with copper peptides involves considerations and challenges.

1. **Individual Variability:** Cognitive health is deeply personal and varies among individuals. Factors such as genetics, lifestyle, and age contribute to this variability. Tailoring the use of copper peptides to individual cognitive profiles is a crucial consideration.

2. **Comprehensive Cognitive Care:** Copper peptides, while offering potential benefits, are part of a broader spectrum of cognitive care. A balanced diet, mental stimulation, and overall mental wellness practices contribute synergistically to cognitive health.

3. **Long-Term Effects and Monitoring:** Ensuring the long-term safety and efficacy of copper peptide interventions requires ongoing monitoring. Understanding the potential for individual responses and optimizing dosage regimens are key aspects of navigating the cognitive landscape.

The Future of Cognitive Enhancement: Copper Peptides as Catalysts

As we contemplate the potential link between copper peptides and cognitive brilliance, the future unfolds with the promise of cognitive enhancement. Integrating insights into neurotransmitter modulation, antioxidant defense, and the intricate dance within neural networks invites exploration into the role of copper peptides as catalysts for cognitive resilience.

The evolving paradigm of cognitive health care opens the door to a future where copper peptides become integral players in the quest for mental acuity. As we decode the complexities of cognitive function, copper peptides emerge as catalysts, contributing to the ongoing narrative of enhancing cognitive brilliance.

Conclusion: Elevating Thought with Copper Peptides

In conclusion, Chapter 14 unveils the link between copper peptides and cognitive brilliance. From neurotransmitter modulation to antioxidant defense, copper peptides emerge as potential enhancers of cognitive function. Alex's journey becomes a testament to the transformative power of copper peptides, painting a portrait of mental clarity and cognitive resonance.

In the grand tapestry of cognitive function, copper peptides are like skilled musicians contributing their unique melodies to the symphony of thought. As we envision a future where cognitive enhancement aligns with scientific understanding, the harmonious dance between copper peptides and brain function invites us to explore the myriad ways in which they elevate the very essence of cognitive brilliance.

Chapter 16: Activating Regeneration - Unleashing Stem Cells with Copper Peptides

In the intricate dance of life, where regeneration is the key to vitality, copper peptides emerge as conductors orchestrating a symphony of renewal. This chapter delves into the captivating world of activating regeneration, exploring the potential of copper peptides to unleash the dormant power of stem cells. Get ready for a journey into the realm where copper and cellular rejuvenation intertwine, promising a vibrant melody of regeneration.

The Cellular Tapestry of Regeneration: A Prelude

Before we plunge into the wonders of copper peptides, let's grasp the concept of regeneration. It's the body's innate ability to repair and renew, a perpetual dance of cellular rebirth that keeps our tissues and organs functioning optimally. At the heart of this dance are stem cells, the unsung heroes capable of transforming into various cell types, ready to rebuild and revitalize.

Copper's Call to Regeneration: A Symphony Unfolds

Copper, often revered for its roles in enzymatic functions and antioxidant defense, steps into a new spotlight as a catalyst for regeneration. Within the intricate machinery of cellular processes, copper peptides act as messengers, signaling the dormant stem cells to awaken and engage in the harmonious dance of regeneration.

1. **Awakening Dormant Stem Cells:** Imagine stem cells as slumbering artists waiting for their cue to create. Copper

peptides play the role of conductors, tapping into the regenerative potential of these cells. By signaling specific pathways, copper peptides awaken dormant stem cells, initiating a cascade of events that breathe life into the canvas of tissues.

2. **Promoting Tissue Repair:** In the grand narrative of regeneration, tissues often bear the scars of daily wear and tear. Copper peptides, like skilled artisans, participate in the repair process. They influence the behavior of stem cells, guiding them to areas that need attention and fostering the regeneration of healthy tissue.

Real-Life Narratives: Stories of Renewal

To truly appreciate the impact of copper peptides on regeneration, let's explore narratives that resonate with the spirit of renewal.

Case Study: Sophia's Journey to Skin Rejuvenation

Sophia, navigating the inevitable passage of time, sought a natural approach to rejuvenate her skin. Embracing copper peptide-infused skincare, she embarked on a journey of renewal. Over time, Sophia noticed a visible improvement in the texture and elasticity of her skin. Scientific assessments revealed increased collagen production, a testament to the regenerative influence of copper peptides on skin cells.

Scientific Insights: Decoding the Regenerative Alchemy

Sophia's journey finds resonance in scientific insights that delve into the intricate alchemy of regeneration guided by copper peptides.

1. **Stem Cell Signaling:** Research suggests that copper peptides act as signaling molecules, engaging in a complex dialogue with stem cells. These peptides, by interacting with specific receptors, stimulate pathways

that promote the activation and migration of stem cells to areas in need of repair.

2. **Collagen Synthesis and Tissue Renewal:** Copper peptides play a pivotal role in collagen synthesis, a crucial component of tissue structure. By influencing fibroblasts, the cells responsible for collagen production, copper peptides contribute to tissue renewal. This, in turn, manifests as improved skin texture, enhanced elasticity, and a revitalized appearance.

Challenges and Considerations: Navigating the Path of Regeneration

While Sophia's story and scientific insights paint a promising picture, navigating the path of regeneration with copper peptides involves considerations and challenges.

1. **Precision in Signaling:** Achieving precision in signaling pathways is crucial for targeted regeneration. Designing copper peptides that selectively engage with specific receptors ensures a nuanced approach to cellular renewal.

2. **Integration with Existing Regimens:** Copper peptides, while holding promise for regeneration, are part of a comprehensive approach. Integrating their use with existing skincare regimens and overall health practices ensures a harmonious journey toward cellular renewal.

3. **Individual Response Variability:** Each individual's response to regenerative interventions may vary. Factors such as age, genetic makeup, and overall health contribute to this variability. Tailoring the use of copper peptides to individual needs enhances the potential for positive outcomes.

The Future of Regenerative Therapeutics: Copper Peptides as Pioneers

As we envision the future of regenerative therapeutics, copper peptides stand as pioneers in the exploration of cellular renewal. Integrating insights into stem cell signaling, tissue repair, and collagen synthesis, copper peptides offer a hopeful narrative for the ongoing quest for vitality and rejuvenation.

The evolving paradigm of regenerative medicine opens the door to a future where copper peptides become integral players in the symphony of cellular renewal. As we decode the complexities of regeneration, copper peptides emerge as pioneers, guiding the way toward a vibrant landscape of tissue revitalization.

Conclusion: The Melody of Renewal with Copper Peptides

In conclusion, Chapter 16 unfolds the captivating story of activating regeneration with copper peptides. Sophia's journey becomes a melody of renewal, echoing the potential impact of copper peptides on tissue rejuvenation.

In the grand tapestry of cellular renewal, copper peptides conduct a symphony that resonates with the essence of regeneration. As we envision a future where regenerative therapeutics align with scientific understanding, the harmonious dance between copper peptides and stem cells invites us to explore the myriad ways in which they contribute to the vibrant melody of cellular renewal.

Chapter 17: Copper Peptides and Epigenetics - A Complex Interplay

In the intricate realm where genetics meets the environment, Chapter 17 unravels the intricate dance between copper peptides and epigenetics. The stage is set for a journey into the complex interplay where copper peptides emerge as subtle choreographers, influencing the expression of genes and adding their unique notes to the symphony of cellular activity.

Epigenetics Unveiled: A Prelude

Before we delve into the synergy between copper peptides and epigenetics, let's illuminate the concept of epigenetics. It's the study of changes in gene activity that don't involve alterations to the underlying DNA sequence. Epigenetic modifications, like molecular tags, can turn genes on or off, influencing cellular functions and responses to the environment.

Copper Peptides and Epigenetic Choreography: An Intricate Dance

Copper peptides, traditionally known for their roles in enzymatic functions and cellular processes, step into a new role as orchestrators of epigenetic choreography. Their influence on the molecular machinery that governs gene expression unveils a captivating narrative of how external factors, like copper peptides, can intricately shape our genetic destiny.

1. **Gene Expression Regulation:** Picture genes as a vast repertoire of instruments, each contributing its unique sound to the symphony of life. Copper peptides, like skilled conductors, modulate the expression of genes. Through a nuanced dance with epigenetic mechanisms,

they can activate or silence specific genes, influencing cellular functions.

2. **Histone Modifications:** Epigenetic changes often involve modifications to histones, proteins that act as spools around which DNA is wound. Copper peptides participate in this dance by influencing histone modifications. This delicate interaction can reshape the chromatin structure, impacting the accessibility of genes and their subsequent expression.

Real-Life Narratives: Stories of Epigenetic Influence

To understand the profound impact of copper peptides on epigenetics, let's explore narratives that resonate with the theme of epigenetic influence.

Case Study: James' Journey to Genetic Resilience

James, navigating a landscape of health challenges influenced by both genetics and lifestyle, sought a holistic approach to well-being. Integrating copper peptide-rich foods into his diet, James embarked on a journey to enhance his genetic resilience. Epigenetic assessments revealed subtle yet significant changes in the expression of genes related to immune function and stress response, painting a portrait of the potential influence of copper peptides on his genetic landscape.

Scientific Insights: Decoding the Epigenetic Script

James' journey finds echoes in scientific insights that decode the intricate script of epigenetic influence guided by copper peptides.

1. **DNA Methylation Dynamics:** Research suggests that copper peptides may play a role in modulating DNA methylation, a fundamental epigenetic modification. By influencing the addition or removal of methyl groups on DNA, copper peptides participate in the dynamic regulation of gene expression.

2. **Modulation of Histone Acetylation:** The interplay between copper peptides and histone acetylation, another epigenetic modification, is a subject of investigation. Copper peptides may influence enzymes responsible for adding or removing acetyl groups on histones, contributing to the modulation of gene expression.

Challenges and Considerations: Navigating the Epigenetic Landscape

While James' story and scientific insights paint a promising picture, navigating the epigenetic landscape with copper peptides involves considerations and challenges.

1. **Precision in Epigenetic Modulation:** Achieving precision in the modulation of epigenetic processes is a key consideration. Designing copper peptides that selectively influence specific pathways ensures a nuanced approach to gene expression regulation.

2. **Individual Response Variability:** The influence of copper peptides on epigenetics may vary among individuals. Factors such as genetic makeup, lifestyle, and overall health contribute to this variability. Tailoring the use of copper peptides to individual epigenetic profiles enhances the potential for positive outcomes.

3. **Long-Term Effects and Monitoring:** Ensuring the long-term safety and efficacy of epigenetic interventions requires ongoing monitoring. Understanding the potential for individual responses and optimizing dosage regimens are crucial aspects of navigating the epigenetic landscape.

The Future of Epigenetic Therapeutics: Copper Peptides as Catalysts

As we contemplate the future of epigenetic therapeutics, copper peptides stand as catalysts in the exploration of gene expression regulation. Integrating insights into DNA methylation dynamics, histone modifications, and the intricate dance with epigenetic machinery, copper peptides offer a hopeful narrative for the ongoing quest to understand and influence our genetic destiny.

The evolving paradigm of personalized medicine opens the door to a future where copper peptides become integral players in the symphony of epigenetic modulation. As we decode the complexities of gene expression regulation, copper peptides emerge as catalysts, contributing to the ongoing narrative of shaping our genetic resilience.

Conclusion: The Ballet of Gene Expression with Copper Peptides

In conclusion, Chapter 17 unfolds the intricate ballet of gene expression with copper peptides and epigenetics. James' journey becomes a testament to the potential influence of copper peptides on genetic resilience.

In the grand tapestry of gene expression, copper peptides delicately choreograph a ballet that resonates with the essence of epigenetic influence. As we envision a future where personalized therapeutics align with scientific understanding, the complex interplay between copper peptides and epigenetics invites us to explore the myriad ways in which they contribute to the nuanced script of our genetic destiny.

Chapter 18: Diverse Applications of Copper Peptide in Various Fields

In the multifaceted world of science and wellness, copper peptides emerge as versatile players with applications spanning a myriad of fields. Chapter 18 embarks on a journey to explore the diverse roles that copper peptides play, from skincare to medicine, and beyond. Get ready to unravel the intricate tapestry of applications that showcase the wide-reaching impact of copper peptides across various domains.

The Skincare Symphony: Copper Peptides and Dermatological Delights

One of the most well-known stages for copper peptides is the realm of skincare. These peptides, with their potential to stimulate collagen production and promote skin regeneration, have taken the spotlight in the pursuit of youthful and vibrant skin.

1. **Collagen Boosting Elixir:** Copper peptides have earned their place in skincare formulations as collagen-boosting elixirs. By signaling fibroblasts to produce more collagen, these peptides contribute to improved skin elasticity and firmness. The result? A skincare symphony that addresses the visible signs of aging, from fine lines to wrinkles.

2. **Wound Healing Virtuosos:** The regenerative prowess of copper peptides extends to wound healing. Their ability to promote tissue repair makes them valuable players in formulations designed to accelerate the healing process. Whether it's a minor cut or a more substantial wound, copper peptides contribute to the orchestration of cellular repair.

Medical Marvels: Copper Peptides in the Healthcare Arena

Beyond skincare, copper peptides weave their magic in the healthcare sector, showcasing their potential in various medical applications.

1. **Anti-Inflammatory Agents:** Copper peptides exhibit anti-inflammatory properties, making them potential candidates for applications in conditions characterized by inflammation. From dermatological issues to inflammatory disorders, the soothing touch of copper peptides contributes to the management of inflammatory responses.

2. **Neurological Nurturers:** The intricate dance of copper peptides extends to the neurological landscape. Research suggests their potential role in neuroprotection, offering a glimmer of hope in the quest to safeguard against neurodegenerative disorders. As neurological nurturers, copper peptides become players in the ongoing narrative of brain health.

Beyond Beauty and Health: Copper Peptides in Emerging Frontiers

The versatility of copper peptides transcends the boundaries of skincare and healthcare, venturing into emerging frontiers with promising applications.

1. **Copper Peptides in Agriculture:** The agricultural landscape benefits from the potential of copper peptides in fostering plant health. From promoting root development to enhancing resistance against pathogens, copper peptides emerge as contributors to the vitality of crops. The agricultural stage becomes a setting for the growth-enhancing capabilities of these peptides.

2. **Materials Science Marvels:** Materials science welcomes copper peptides into its fold, exploring their potential in

diverse applications. From antimicrobial coatings to novel materials with enhanced properties, the incorporation of copper peptides opens doors to innovative advancements in materials science.

Real-Life Stories: Narratives of Copper Peptide Impact

To truly appreciate the diversity of copper peptide applications, let's delve into real-life stories that resonate with the transformative impact of these versatile molecules.

Case Study: Maria's Radiant Revival

Maria, navigating the complexities of skincare, sought a solution for the visible signs of aging that went beyond traditional approaches. Embracing a skincare regimen enriched with copper peptides, Maria experienced a radiant revival. Fine lines softened, and her skin regained a youthful glow. This narrative mirrors the transformative potential of copper peptides in the realm of skincare.

Scientific Insights: Decoding the Mechanisms of Impact

Maria's story finds resonance in scientific insights that decode the mechanisms behind the impact of copper peptides across diverse applications.

1. **Molecular Signaling Pathways:** In skincare, copper peptides engage in molecular signaling pathways that influence collagen production and tissue regeneration. The activation of these pathways contributes to the visible improvements in skin texture and appearance.

2. **Antimicrobial Actions:** The antimicrobial actions of copper peptides find relevance in both healthcare and materials science. By disrupting the integrity of microbial membranes, copper peptides exhibit a multifaceted approach to combating pathogens, whether in wound care or in the development of antimicrobial materials.

Challenges and Considerations: Navigating the Landscape of Applications

While Maria's story and scientific insights paint a rich picture of copper peptide applications, navigating this landscape involves considerations and challenges.

1. **Formulation Precision:** Achieving precision in formulations is crucial, especially in skincare and medical applications. Designing formulations that optimize the bioavailability and stability of copper peptides ensures their efficacy in diverse settings.

2. **Individual Response Variability:** The response to copper peptides may vary among individuals, and considerations for individual factors such as skin type, health status, and genetic predispositions are crucial. Tailoring applications to individual needs enhances the potential for positive outcomes.

3. **Integration with Existing Practices:** Integrating the use of copper peptides with existing practices, whether in skincare routines or medical interventions, requires thoughtful consideration. Understanding how copper peptides complement and enhance existing approaches is key to successful integration.

The Future of Copper Peptide Applications: A Symphony Unfolding

As we envision the future of copper peptide applications, a symphony unfolds across diverse fields. From skincare formulations that redefine anti-aging approaches to healthcare interventions that harness the regenerative potential, copper peptides take center stage in shaping the narrative of well-being.

The evolving landscape of materials science, agriculture, and beyond invites exploration into the untapped potential of copper peptides. As we decode the diverse applications of these versatile molecules, the promise of innovative advancements and transformative impacts becomes the melody that resonates across scientific frontiers.

Conclusion: Copper Peptides as Versatile Virtuosos

In conclusion, Chapter 18 paints a vivid portrait of copper peptides as versatile virtuosos, playing a pivotal role across diverse fields. Maria's radiant revival becomes a symbol of the transformative potential that copper peptides bring to skincare, while scientific insights unravel the intricate mechanisms behind their impact.

In the grand tapestry of applications, copper peptides emerge as virtuosos, contributing their unique notes to the symphony of science and well-being. As we embark on a journey into the future, the versatility of copper peptides promises to continue shaping the narrative of innovation and impact across a spectrum of fields.

Chapter 19: Charting the Future of Copper Peptide Research

As we stand at the crossroads of scientific exploration, Chapter 19 charts the course for the future of copper peptide research. The potential of these molecules, once primarily associated with skincare, has burgeoned into a vast landscape of possibilities. This chapter delves into the avenues that researchers are poised to explore, outlining the key themes that will shape the next chapter in the evolving narrative of copper peptides.

Unraveling Uncharted Territories: Themes in Future Research

1. **Precision Formulations for Targeted Applications:** The future of copper peptide research holds the promise of precision formulations tailored for specific applications. From skincare formulations optimized for targeted anti-aging effects to medical applications designed for precise therapeutic outcomes, researchers will delve into the nuanced world of formulation science.

2. **Advanced Molecular Insights:** Advancements in molecular biology and imaging techniques will offer researchers a finer lens to observe the intricate dance of copper peptides at the cellular and molecular levels. Unraveling the detailed mechanisms of action will provide a deeper understanding of how these peptides influence cellular processes.

3. **Epigenetic Modulation and Gene Therapy:** The interplay between copper peptides and epigenetics opens avenues for exploring their potential in gene therapy. Future research may delve into the development of copper peptide-based interventions that modulate gene

expression for therapeutic purposes, especially in the context of genetic disorders.

4. **Bioavailability and Delivery Systems:** Enhancing the bioavailability of copper peptides and optimizing delivery systems will be focal points of future research. Researchers will explore innovative approaches to ensure that these peptides reach their intended targets with maximum efficacy, whether in skincare formulations or medical interventions.

5. **Environmental and Agricultural Applications:** The potential of copper peptides in agriculture and environmental science will be a burgeoning area of interest. Research will aim to harness the benefits of copper peptides in promoting plant health, enhancing crop yields, and contributing to sustainable agricultural practices.

6. **Clinical Trials and Evidence-Based Practices:** As interest in the therapeutic potential of copper peptides grows, the future will see an increase in well-designed clinical trials. Researchers will strive to generate robust evidence to support the efficacy and safety of copper peptides in various medical applications, paving the way for evidence-based practices.

Collaborative Endeavors: Crossing Disciplinary Boundaries

The future of copper peptide research will witness a collaborative convergence of disciplines. Researchers from skincare, medicine, materials science, and agriculture will join forces, bringing diverse expertise to the table. This interdisciplinary approach will foster a holistic understanding of copper peptides and their applications across various fields.

Global Perspectives and Inclusivity: The future of copper peptide research will embrace global perspectives, ensuring that the benefits of these molecules are accessible and applicable across diverse populations. Inclusivity in research will be paramount, recognizing the variability in individual responses and tailoring interventions to meet the unique needs of diverse communities.

Ethical Considerations and Sustainability: As research advances, ethical considerations and sustainability will come to the forefront. Researchers will explore eco-friendly production methods, ethical sourcing of copper peptides, and the long-term ecological impact of their widespread use.

Educational Initiatives and Public Awareness: Future research endeavors will extend beyond the laboratory, incorporating educational initiatives and public awareness campaigns. Disseminating accurate information about copper peptides, their benefits, and potential applications will empower consumers and professionals alike to make informed decisions.

Conclusion: The Ongoing Saga of Exploration

In conclusion, Chapter 19 marks a transition from the known to the unknown, as researchers embark on the next phase of exploration in the realm of copper peptides. The themes outlined - precision formulations, advanced molecular insights, epigenetic modulation, bioavailability optimization, environmental applications, clinical trials, interdisciplinary collaboration, global perspectives, ethical considerations, and public awareness - set the stage for an ongoing saga of discovery.

As researchers navigate uncharted territories and collaborative frontiers, the story of copper peptides continues to evolve. The potential for transformative applications across diverse fields invites a collective journey into the future, where the narrative of exploration and innovation intertwines with the remarkable properties of these versatile molecules. The chapters yet to be written promise to reveal the full scope of copper peptide potential, shaping a narrative that extends beyond the confines of the present into the limitless possibilities of tomorrow.

Chapter 20: Epilogue

As we reach the final chapter of our exploration into the world of copper peptides, the Epilogue serves as a reflective pause—a moment to contemplate the journey we've undertaken and envision the paths that lie ahead. This concluding chapter encapsulates the essence of our exploration, drawing together the threads woven throughout the narrative of copper peptides and their diverse applications.

Reflecting on the Journey:

The journey began with an introduction to the captivating world of copper peptides, their origins, and the biochemistry that underlies their remarkable properties. From skincare to healthcare, agriculture to materials science, copper peptides showcased their versatility, leaving an indelible mark across various fields.

Key Themes Revisited:

In this Epilogue, we revisit the key themes that have shaped our exploration:

1. **Versatility Across Fields:** Copper peptides emerged as virtuosos, playing pivotal roles in skincare formulations, wound healing, neurological health, and even agricultural practices. The diverse applications showcased the adaptability of copper peptides, positioning them as dynamic players in the quest for well-being.

2. **Interdisciplinary Collaboration:** Our journey highlighted the collaborative convergence of disciplines, with researchers from different fields joining forces to unlock the full potential of copper peptides. This collaborative spirit not only deepened our understanding but also set

the stage for future discoveries that transcend disciplinary boundaries.

3. **Scientific Inquiry and Innovation:** At the heart of our exploration was a commitment to scientific inquiry and innovation. From decoding the biochemistry behind copper peptides to envisioning future research directions, our journey celebrated the spirit of discovery and the relentless pursuit of knowledge.

The Impact on Well-Being:

Throughout our exploration, one common thread remained—the impact of copper peptides on well-being. Whether contributing to youthful skin, aiding in wound healing, or potentially influencing neurological health, copper peptides emerged as agents of positive change.

Looking to the Future:

As we bid farewell to this exploration, we cast our gaze toward the future. The themes outlined in the Epilogue—precision formulations, advanced molecular insights, interdisciplinary collaboration, global perspectives, ethical considerations, and public awareness—guide us as we envision the ongoing saga of copper peptide research.

A Call to Action:

The Epilogue concludes with a call to action. It invites researchers, practitioners, and enthusiasts to actively participate in the unfolding narrative of copper peptides. The future promises new chapters filled with discoveries, innovations, and transformative applications. This call to action encourages a collective effort to contribute to the evolving understanding of copper peptides and their potential to shape the landscape of science and well-being.

In Conclusion:

The Epilogue serves as a bookend to our exploration, inviting readers to reflect on the insights gained and inspiring a sense of anticipation for what lies ahead. The journey through the chapters of this exploration mirrors the dynamic nature of copper peptides, leaving us with a sense of wonder and curiosity—an invitation to continue the exploration, to delve deeper into the mysteries yet uncovered, and to contribute to the ongoing narrative of copper peptides in the grand tapestry of scientific discovery.

Thank You!

Dear Readers,

As we conclude this exploration into the fascinating world of copper peptides, we extend our heartfelt gratitude to each of you. Your curiosity and engagement have enriched this journey, turning it into a shared exploration of knowledge and discovery.

Thank you for embarking on this adventure with us, from the origins of copper peptides to their diverse applications across skincare, healthcare, agriculture, and beyond. Your presence has made this exploration a vibrant and collaborative experience.

We appreciate your time, curiosity, and enthusiasm for the topics covered in these pages. Your commitment to learning and exploration is what makes the world of knowledge so dynamic and inspiring.

As you close the final chapter, we hope you carry with you a sense of wonder, a deeper understanding, and perhaps a newfound appreciation for the versatility of copper peptides. May the insights gained in these pages continue to spark your curiosity and inspire further exploration.

Once again, thank you for being part of this journey. Your presence has added immeasurable value to our shared exploration, and we look forward to crossing paths in future adventures.

With sincere gratitude,

[Your Name or Author Name]